Annabel Karmel
Eating for Two

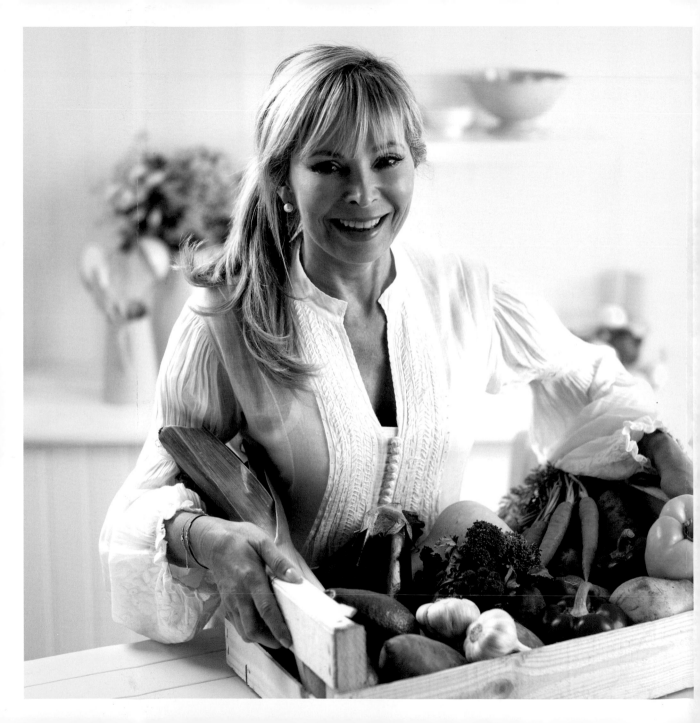

Annabel Karmel
Eating for Two

The complete guide to nutrition during pregnancy and beyond

Consultant Dietitian/Nutritionist:
Fiona Hinton, BSc, MNutDiet, RD

ATRIA BOOKS

New York • London • Toronto • Sydney • New Delhi

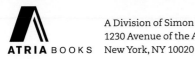

A Division of Simon & Schuster, Inc.
1230 Avenue of the Americas
New York, NY 10020

Originally published in 2012 by Ebury Press, an imprint of Ebury Publishing,
a Random House Group Company

First Atria Books hardcover edition August 2013

ATRIA B O O K S and colophon are trademarks of Simon & Schuster, Inc.

For information about special discounts for bulk purchases,
please contact Simon & Schuster Special Sales at
1-866-506-1949 or business@simonandschuster.com.

The Simon & Schuster Speakers Bureau can bring authors
to your live event. For more information or to book an event,
contact the Simon & Schuster Speakers Bureau at
1-866-248-3049 or visit our website at www.simonspeakers.com.

Manufactured in China

10 9 8 7 6 5 4 3 2 1

Library of Congress Cataloging-in-Publication data is available.

ISBN 978-1-4767-2975-6
ISBN 978-1-4767-2977-0 (ebook)

Contents

1: Good Nutrition: The Building Blocks for Your Baby

Why good nutrition is crucial during pregnancy

Welcome to the most amazing time of your life. Your body is beginning a fantastic roller-coaster ride, and while the ups and downs of pregnancy may be a mix of the joyful, the amusing, and even the downright unpleasant, this is a journey that will remain with you forever. Good nutrition has a huge influence on pregnancy, both for mom and for baby. It's one of the first gifts we can give our child.

We all want the best for our babies, and eating a balanced and nutritious diet during pregnancy helps to give them an optimal start in life in a number of different ways. A steady supply of vitamins, minerals, protein, and other nutrients is crucial to an unborn baby's development. It allows the mother to form a healthy placenta, the baby's lifeline from the outside world. A healthy diet also allows the baby to lay down stores of nutrients, such as iron, that will be necessary during the first months of life outside the uterus.

We often focus so much on babies that we forget the importance of these nutrients for mom; they're essential to support changes such as the growth of the placenta and uterus. At the end of pregnancy, it is essential for the body to be well nourished to cope with the demands of labor and breast-feeding.

One great advantage of a healthy diet is that it allows both mother and baby to gain a healthy amount of weight. This has benefits both during pregnancy and the birth, as well as when mother and baby begin their new life together, and beyond.

Giving your baby the best start in life begins now, whether you are planning to become pregnant, have just found out the happy news, or have a bump well on the way. Start with "First priorities," below, then read on to find out about foods to focus on, how to tackle nutritional problems, and delicious recipes tailored to each trimester.

First priorities

If you're like most new moms-to-be, your brain probably started racing as soon as you found out you were pregnant. Trying to process myriad thoughts, from baby names to the birth, can make it difficult to remember what to do first. So here's a list of the very first actions to take to benefit both your health and that of your baby. None of these actions is difficult to carry out, and the sooner you start, the sooner you'll be putting your own and your baby's well-being at the top of your priority list.

Start taking folic acid and vitamin D

While there's a lot of information on vitamins and minerals in this book, the first ones to think about, as early as possible in your pregnancy or even beforehand, are folic acid and vitamin D. Taking supplements of folic acid, a B vitamin, has been shown to reduce the risk of the unborn baby's

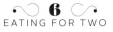

developing spina bifida and other neural tube defects (types of malformation in the baby's spinal cord). Start taking 400 mcg (micrograms) of folic acid daily from before conception or as early as possible in the pregnancy, and continue until the end of the first trimester. The recommendation is higher—5,000 mcg (5 mg) of folic acid per day—if you have had a previous pregnancy or are yourself affected by a neural tube defect, are taking epilepsy medication, or have diabetes, celiac disease, thalassemia, or sickle-cell anemia; speak to your ob-gyn for further advice. Also, try to eat some foods rich in folic acid every day. These include breakfast cereals with added folic acid, yeast extract, oranges and orange juice, and green leafy vegetables.

Recent studies have shown that more people have low vitamin D levels than was previously thought. While foods such as fortified margarines, oil-rich fish, and eggs contain some vitamin D, the main source is the action of strong sunlight on the skin. Because this also carries risks, keep to moderate sun exposure (you don't need to sunbathe) and take a daily supplement of 10 mcg of vitamin D during your pregnancy and if and when you are breast-feeding.

You can read more about folic acid and vitamin D later in this chapter (see page 16).

Think before you drink
Authorities are divided on whether it's safe to drink a small amount of alcohol while you're pregnant or whether to avoid even the tiniest amount. The current advice from the UK's National Health Service (NHS) and the United States Surgeon General is not to drink alcohol at all while pregnant.

If you do, keep it to a small occasional drink, and only after the first trimester. Your baby is most vulnerable during the first trimester when crucial development is taking place. Read more about drinking alcohol during pregnancy on page 29.

Think before you eat
By reading this book, you'll gain a wealth of information on feeding yourself (and therefore also your baby) as well as possible during your pregnancy. If you think before you eat, you can focus on foods that provide essential protein, vitamins, and other nutrients, which are the building blocks for your developing baby. You can also avoid eating too many "empty calories"—foods that are high in calories from fat or sugar, but not high in nutrients. This helps to prevent too much weight gain, which can cause problems for both you and your baby. Lastly, thinking about what you eat, and how it's prepared and stored, can help to minimize the risk of food poisoning and other food-related issues during pregnancy.

Dodge the smoke
It goes without saying that if cigarette smoke is unhealthy for us, it will be unhealthy for our unborn babies. Research has found that smoking during pregnancy is associated with a higher risk of problems, ranging from babies being born early to miscarriage. If you are a smoker, speak to your ob-gyn about strategies to help you cut down or quit. This may even reduce your morning sickness. If you are not a smoker, be aware of secondhand smoke, which is also related to problems such as lower birth weight for babies.

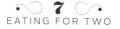

Review your pills and potions

It's easy to continue to take your usual medications or supplements when you become pregnant, just out of habit. However, this is not a time to take any nonessential pills or potions, even nutritional supplements or herbal remedies. Essential medications should also be reviewed for safety during pregnancy and possible alternatives prescribed. Whether prescription or over-the-counter, discuss all your medication needs with your pharmacist or ob-gyn.

How much weight should I gain?

Gaining an appropriate amount of weight is critical during pregnancy. The weight of the baby is about 7 to 8 pounds, but you are also gaining a placenta through which to pass nutrients to your baby, the amniotic fluid he is swimming in, larger breasts, and so on. You might think it would take a huge amount of extra calories to achieve all this, but actually it's more a case of quality rather than quantity. You are most certainly "eating for two" because there are now two of you whose well-being is dependent on what you eat, and because pregnancy increases your requirement for a host of nutrients. However, you actually don't require extra calories until the last trimester of pregnancy, and even then it's quite a small increase (see page 120).

There are risks associated with gaining too much weight—these include a higher chance of having a larger baby and a more difficult labor. The risks can be long term; research has found that mothers who gain more weight than recommended during pregnancy are more likely to be overweight many years later. On the other side of the coin, gaining too little weight during pregnancy may increase the risk of having a smaller baby and a premature birth.

Amazing as it may seem, there's also increasing concern among some scientists that the quality of a pregnant woman's diet, as well as the amount of weight gain during pregnancy, could affect her child's health many years, even many decades, later. For example, babies receiving very poor nutrition during the pregnancy, or being born with a low birth weight and then growing quickly to "catch up," seem to be at increased risk of being overweight or developing heart disease as an adult. Babies born with a high birth weight also have an increased risk of being overweight, both as children and as adults.

While British authorities don't issue an actual guideline on weight gain, they suggest that the usual weight gain during pregnancy is about 22 to 28 pounds, with most of this gained after twenty weeks. In the United States and Canada, health authorities do have more detailed guidelines: For women who begin their pregnancy within their healthy weight range, they recommend a weight gain of 25 to 35 pounds. This is made up of 2.2 to 4.4 pounds total weight gain during the first trimester, and about 1 pound on average per week after that.

This changes if you are over- or underweight to start with. For moms-to-be who are below the healthy weight range when they become pregnant, the guideline is to gain 28 to 40 pounds. If you are overweight, with a BMI between 25 and 29.9, the goal is 15 to 25 pounds; if your BMI is over 30, the guidelines suggest you limit weight gain to 11 to 20 pounds.

If you are expecting twins, the U.S. and Canadian authorities recommend a weight gain of 37 to 55 pounds if you begin pregnancy within the healthy weight range. I suggest that if you are expecting more than two babies, or are over- or underweight at the beginning of your pregnancy, you ask your ob-gyn for further guidance on how much weight you should gain.

In reality, if you eat to satisfy your appetite and follow a balanced diet, your weight gain is likely to be within the recommended amounts. However, some moms-to-be find it difficult to eat enough due to morning sickness, or because they feel very full in the third trimester. Others may find that their appetite increases dramatically in the second trimester and they have trouble resisting the little extras that can lead to excess weight gain. See the sections on each trimester for more on these issues.

What's my pre-pregnancy BMI?

While many of us can tell just by looking in the mirror whether we are over- or underweight, the way doctors tell is by calculating our body mass index (BMI). You can calculate it yourself, but there are many BMI calculators on the Internet. (Calculate BMI by dividing weight in pounds by height in inches squared, then multiplying by a conversion factor of 703. Internet charts are a lot easier!)

If your BMI is between 18.5 and 24.9, you are within your healthy weight range. Any higher or lower and you are over- or underweight and your recommended weight gain during pregnancy changes accordingly.

Where does all the weight go?

It can be mystifying to gain 29 pounds, yet give birth to an 8-pound baby. Here's a guide to where the other pounds go:

Your baby: about 7 to 8 pounds
Your blossoming breasts: about 2.2 pounds
Your growing uterus: about 2.2 pounds
The placenta: about 1.5 pounds
The amniotic fluid: about 2.2 pounds
Increased blood volume: about 3 to 4 pounds
Increased fluid volume: about 3 to 4 pounds
Laying down fat stores (in preparation for
    breast-feeding): about 6 to 8 pounds

Remember, an unborn baby is most vulnerable in the first months after conception, so this is the most important time to follow a healthy diet, rather than restrict your intake. This includes the time when you don't yet know you're pregnant. Eating well is the most important priority at the time of conception, for your baby's short- and long-term health. And if you are planning to make changes to your diet or take supplements while trying to conceive, discuss it with your ob-gyn first to be sure you are not taking any risks with your health or that of your baby.

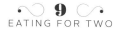

Nutrition ABCs

Start with the basics

We really are what we eat—a healthy diet promotes a healthy body and a healthy baby. The reason for this comes down to the building blocks that make up our food, and if we understand them, it makes it easier to understand how best to build our diet. And while the easiest way to plan your diet is using the food groups, it's the substances within those groups—the protein, vitamins, and fiber, for example—that make each one important.

Pregnancy Myth Buster: Special diets for boys and girls

Many parents-to-be have a secret yearning for either a baby blue or a pastel pink delivery, and you may be bombarded with suggestions of how to conceive either a boy or a girl. Many of these involve people changing their diets before they conceive, from eating a lot of acidic foods, such as oranges, to eating higher-potassium foods, such as bananas, to taking extra magnesium supplements. Some theories are really just old wives' tales, though others do have some basis in scientific research. A 2008 study found that mothers eating a higher-calorie diet that contained more breakfast cereals before they became pregnant had slightly more boys than girls, compared with mothers eating a lower-calorie diet. However, the change in odds of having one sex over the other was slight. For example, 9 out of 20 of the women following the higher-calorie diet had girls, compared with 11 having boys. Most important, the mothers eating a higher-calorie diet were also eating a better-quality diet, with higher levels of vitamins and minerals, so also giving their babies the best start in life.

Protein

A major component of muscle, protein also forms hormones and a host of other substances. In total, protein makes up about a fifth of the body's tissues (excluding fat), which makes a healthy protein intake integral to your baby's development as well as to your body's growth during pregnancy.

Protein is made up of building blocks called amino acids, and we need to obtain a range of these amino acids from our diet to form the protein in our bodies. Many people think of meat as our main protein source. In fact, meat, poultry, and fish are very rich in high-quality protein, as are dairy foods and eggs—this means they supply all the amino acids required in a balance appropriate to the body's needs. Many plant foods also contain significant amounts of protein, including soy, dried beans, lentils, and other legumes; nuts; seeds; mycoprotein; and grain foods. The difference is that, apart from soy and quinoa, no major plant foods contain protein of a similar amino-acid profile to animal foods. However, if you eat a combination of plant food types over a day, such as toast at breakfast, lentil soup for lunch, and a nutty stir-fry with rice for your evening meal, your overall intake will provide a balance of all amino acids. This means vegetarians and vegans can easily meet their protein needs just by eating a varied diet.

Carbohydrates

Carbohydrates (or carbs) have almost become dirty words in the last few years, receiving more than their share of blame for people becoming overweight. In fact, they are an essential part of a healthy diet, as long as they are chosen wisely.

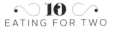

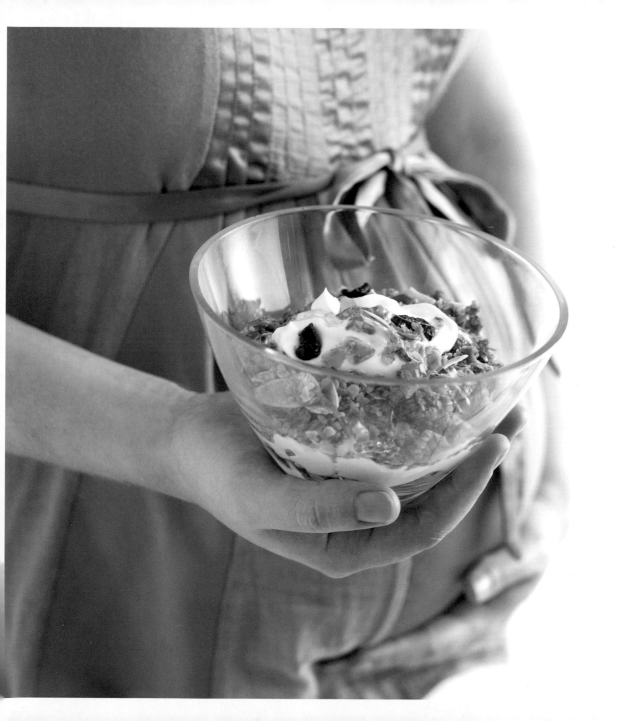

Carbohydrates are the sugars and starches in our food, and they are also our body's main fuel supply, a bit like the gasoline that fuels a car. As your baby grows, the carbohydrates in your diet will also become her fuel supply. It's better to focus on the starchy rather than the sugary types; starchy carbohydrates are found mainly in grain foods such as bread, breakfast cereal, rice, and pasta, as well as in potatoes.

Fruit is a healthy source of sugars, but the sugars in sweet foods, such as sugary drinks, candy, sugary breakfast cereals, and cookies, should be kept to a minimum.

Try to choose higher-fiber carbohydrate foods, such as whole grains, and leave the skins on fruits and potatoes where possible. You can read more about fiber, and about low-glycemic-index carbs, which may keep your body fueled for longer, in chapter 3 (see page 71).

Fat

Like carbs, fat has also become a dreaded substance in recent years. While eating too many of the wrong sorts of fat is undeniably unhealthy, fats also serve functions such as carrying certain vitamins from the intestine into the body, insulating people from the cold, and forming part of the membrane around all cells in the body. Many people don't realize that some types of fat are essential to our bodies and crucial to a baby's development during pregnancy. Everyone should minimize the saturated fat (from meat fat, the skin on poultry, dairy foods, and processed foods that contain coconut and palm oils) and trans fats (from processed foods

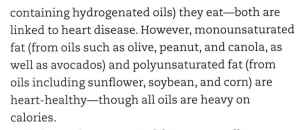

containing hydrogenated oils) they eat—both are linked to heart disease. However, monounsaturated fat (from oils such as olive, peanut, and canola, as well as avocados) and polyunsaturated fat (from oils including sunflower, soybean, and corn) are heart-healthy—though all oils are heavy on calories.

In fact, polyunsaturated fats are actually essential. For example, they are needed for the formation of a range of substances that regulate body processes, such as immune function and blood clotting. They are made up of two types: omega-3 and omega-6. Both of these fats are particularly important during pregnancy because they are required for the formation of brain, nerve, and eye tissue in your developing baby. The need is especially high during the rapid growth of the third trimester.

While both types are essential, it's the omega-3 fats you need to concentrate on, because people generally eat more omega-6 than they require from their usual diet. Most people don't eat enough omega-3, however, and during pregnancy and breast-feeding, it's especially important. Omega-3s may sound familiar because the main source is the healthy fish oils we hear so much about. This is the reason why we are advised to eat two servings of fish each week, at least one of which is an oil-rich fish. These include fresh and canned salmon and mackerel, and fresh tuna. There are, however, restrictions on the types and amounts of fish that can be eaten during pregnancy—you can read more about this on page 27. Obtaining omega-3 oils becomes more difficult if you don't or can't eat fish. A different version of omega-3 oil is found in some

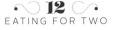

plant foods, including walnuts, flaxseed (also called linseed), and oil made from them. The problem is that the body converts only a small amount of the omega-3 from plants to the type found in fish, which is the type needed by the body. Certain fish oil supplements are not recommended in pregnancy because some are high in vitamin A (see page 26), but if you don't eat fish, you might like to discuss omega-3-supplement options with your ob-gyn. Some are made from algae, so are suitable for vegans. You can find more information in Pregnancy Supernutrients (page 16).

Vitamins and minerals

There is a huge range of vitamins and minerals that are essential to our bodies (and our babies), though in very small amounts. Those that are especially critical during pregnancy include iron, calcium, folic acid, and vitamin D. You can read more about these in Pregnancy Supernutrients (page 16). For the others, please rest assured that a balanced diet as outlined in the "Following the food groups" section will more than meet your needs.

Fiber

Fiber is the part of food that does not get absorbed on its way through the body, but passes straight through you. Fiber is found only in plant foods, including grains, fruit and vegetables, seeds, nuts, and legumes such as dried peas and beans, lentils, and chickpeas. While fiber brings a range of health benefits, during pregnancy a major role is helping to prevent constipation. To increase fiber intake, choose whole-grain foods; enjoy dried fruits, nuts, and seeds; eat fruits and vegetables unpeeled where possible; and eat legumes in the form of lentil soup, baked beans, and bean salad. You can read more about fiber and constipation on page 72.

Following the food groups

Yes, I know: You've read all about the food groups before. This time it's different, though; this time you're pregnant and your baby's well-being and development depend on it. So take the time for a little revision. It's useful for you and your baby right now, but you'll also need to think about food groups when breast-feeding and weaning your baby.

About a third of the total food you eat should come from bread, other grain foods, and potatoes. These are an important fuel supply for your body, and you should base your meals around them. About another third should come from fruit and vegetables. Aim for at least five servings of these a day—Pregnancy Supernutrients gives you a guideline as to what makes up one serving. Try to choose a range of colors of fruit and vegetables, rather than relying on the same choices each day. Also aim to choose mainly higher-fiber options, meaning whole-grain rather than "white" grain foods, and fruit or vegetables in a more "whole" state, leaving the skin on where possible and limiting juice to one of the five servings. Skipping higher-sugar and higher-fat grain foods, such as croissants, cookies, and pastries, will also ensure healthier choices, as will limiting the amount of butter or spread you use.

Both milk and dairy foods as well as meat, fish, and vegetarian alternatives (including eggs, beans, tofu, lentils, and nuts) are valuable sources of

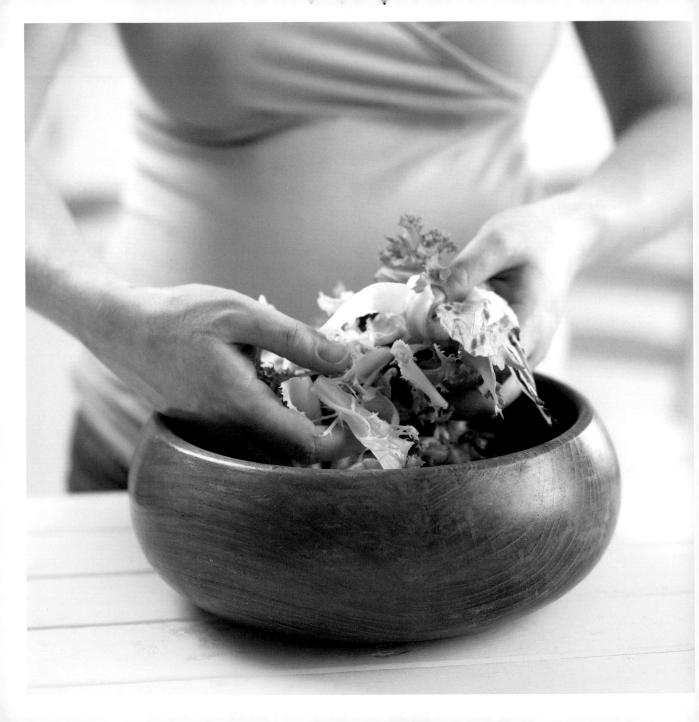

protein. In addition, the dairy foods supply bone-building calcium, and meat and alternatives are generally rich in iron, a nutrient that can run short during pregnancy. Despite their importance, smaller amounts are required from these food groups: 2 or 3 servings per day from dairy foods (though this rockets to 4 or 5 per day during breast-feeding) and about 2 per day from meat, fish, and alternatives. Again, look for lower-fat options, so trim the fat off meat and the skin off chicken, choose reduced-fat dairy foods, and cook by roasting, broiling, or baking rather than frying. Note that if you do not eat dairy foods, you can choose calcium-fortified soy milks and desserts as an alternative. For more on this, see the information on calcium on page 18.

There is a small allowance for higher-fat and higher-sugar foods. You don't need to eat perfectly all the time, but aim to keep foods such as cake, pastries, candy, soda, fries, and chips to an occasional treat. As well as supplying unnecessary calories, they contain very little of the nutrients you and your baby need at this critical time. Instead, you could try some of the "naughty (but still nutritious)" treats listed on page 124.

Fruit and vegetables: Aim for at least five servings each day, whether fresh, frozen, canned, dried, or juice. One serving equals:
* 1 piece of fruit such as an apple, pear, or orange
* 1 large slice of melon or pineapple
* 3 heaping tablespoons of vegetables
* 3 heaping tablespoons of canned fruit
* 1 bowl of salad
* 1 small glass of pure juice

Bread, other grain foods, and potatoes: Base your meals around these foods. They include bread and rolls, English muffins, wraps, breakfast cereal, rice, pasta, and potatoes. Opt for whole-grain foods where possible.

Meat, poultry, fish, eggs, and alternatives: These foods should make up about one-sixth of the food you eat. Eat about 2 servings per day. Try to include 2 servings of fish per week, including at least 1 serving of oil-rich fish.

Milk and dairy: Eat 2 or 3 servings per day, looking for reduced-fat options. One serving equals:
* 1 glass milk
* 1 cup yogurt
* 1 ounce cheese (about the size of a matchbox)

High-fat and high-sugar foods: Limit these to small amounts or an occasional treat.

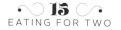

Pregnancy Supernutrients

All nutrients are critical during pregnancy because all are required to build a healthy baby (and keep you healthy as well). Most of us have sufficient amounts of some nutrients, such as vitamin A, from our diet and stored in our bodies already, so even though there is an increased requirement for vitamin A during pregnancy, there is very little risk of not getting enough (and there are risks associated with consuming too much; see page 26). With other nutrients, such as iron and vitamin D, there is a higher risk of not getting enough; therefore, you need to be more mindful of your diet to ensure you do meet your needs, or to take a supplement when necessary. Here are eight key nutrients to keep in mind while you're pregnant, and while breast-feeding.

Supernutrient: FOLIC ACID

Importance: Research has shown that an increased intake of folic acid (a B vitamin) during early pregnancy dramatically reduces the risk of a baby's having a neural tube defect (a type of spine malformation), such as spina bifida. Folic acid also plays a pivotal role in cell division, so is vital throughout pregnancy for your baby's development. In addition, a study has found that women who took folic acid supplements for a year before becoming pregnant had a lower risk of premature labor. For this, and because many women become pregnant without planning to, some experts have called for all women of childbearing age to take folic acid supplements all the time.

Intake: As well as maximizing intake by regularly eating the foods listed below, it's recommended that women take a 400 mcg folic acid supplement daily before conception (if possible) and during the first trimester of pregnancy. For women with a family history of neural tube defects, or with certain chronic health problems, the recommendation is increased to 5,000 mcg per day (5 mg per day).

Where to find it: Sources of folic acid include:

* Breakfast cereals or breads with added folic acid (check the label to be sure)
* Yeast extract
* Citrus fruits and juices
* Legumes
* Green leafy vegetables, including brussels sprouts, kale, broccoli, and spinach
* Peas
* Bananas
* Asparagus

Note that foods must be eaten raw or very lightly cooked, otherwise folic acid is destroyed.

Supernutrient: IRON

Importance: Iron intake becomes more important during pregnancy for a number of reasons: Firstly, it is a component of the baby's and mother's red blood cells. Red blood cells are being manufactured by the growing baby, but pregnant women also increase their blood volume by about 20 percent. Iron is also required for placental development, and

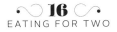

the metabolism of both mother and baby. During the third trimester, iron requirements increase even more because babies are laying down iron stores to last them through the first six months after birth. Thus, iron deficiency is quite common during pregnancy (see page 122).

Intake: While there is no recommendation for an increased iron intake during pregnancy (partly because pregnant women absorb more iron), it's important to eat iron-rich foods regularly.

Where to find it: An easily absorbed form of iron is found in red meat, with smaller amounts in poultry and fish (particularly dark meat and oil-rich fish), including canned crab.

Plant-based foods and eggs contain iron that is not so easily absorbed. Sources include:

* Fortified breakfast cereal
* Eggs
* Fortified white and whole wheat bread
* Green leafy vegetables, such as spinach
* Legumes
* Soybean flour
* Dried fruit, such as apricots
* Wheat germ
* Nuts and seeds

The absorption of this form of iron is enhanced by eating a food containing vitamin C, or by eating meat or poultry at the same time. If your iron stores are low, try to avoid dairy foods, tea, and coffee with meals—they all block iron absorption.

Note that liver is very high in iron, but it should not be eaten during pregnancy because it's also high in vitamin A, an excess of which can cause malformations in the baby.

Supernutrient: OMEGA-3 FATS

Importance: These are the fats found in oil-rich fish. They are a major component of brain, eye, and nerve tissue, and are therefore critical to the development of your growing baby. The baby's brain continues developing after birth, so keeping up the supply is vital if you're breast-feeding. There may also be other benefits: Research suggests that unborn babies "fed" sufficient omega-3s have a higher IQ as young children, and that mothers eating sufficient amounts may have a lower incidence of postpartum depression.

Intake: It's recommended that you eat oil-rich fish once or twice a week, with a serving size of about 3.5 to 5 ounces. Note the limitations on the amount and types of fish that should be eaten during pregnancy (see page 27).

Where to find it: Oil-rich fish include salmon, tuna, trout, herring, mackerel, sardines, and canned versions of any but tuna. "Omega-3-rich eggs" from chickens fed a special diet to boost the omega-3 content of their eggs contain smaller amounts of this type of fat.

Even in limited amounts, fish is by far the best source of omega-3s. If you don't or can't eat fish, you can get small amounts of plant-based omega-3 oils from a number of foods. Unfortunately, only a small amount of these are converted in the body to the fish-oil-type omega-3 that we need. Plant sources include:

* Walnuts and walnut oil
* Flaxseed (also called linseed) and flaxseed oil
* Canola oil (cold-pressed, if possible)
* Soy foods
* Some green vegetables, such as arugula and broccoli

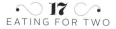

If you are thinking about taking a fish oil supplement, make sure it's not a fish liver oil because they can be high in vitamin A. Vegans might consider an omega-3 supplement made from algae. Always discuss with your ob-gyn.

Supernutrient: CALCIUM

Importance: Calcium is a building block of your developing baby's bones and teeth, most of it laid down in the last ten weeks of pregnancy. Thus it is a mineral we need to be aware of during pregnancy (and even more while breast-feeding, because a lot is lost through breast milk). While the requirement during pregnancy doesn't increase, because your body cleverly increases the amount it absorbs from your diet, calcium intake can be an issue for people who don't consume dairy products.

Intake: Aim to eat 2 or 3 servings of dairy food per day while pregnant, and more while breast-feeding. See page 15 for serving sizes.

Where to find it: The best source of calcium is dairy foods, including milk, cheese, and yogurt. The absorption of calcium is also enhanced by the presence of vitamin D.

If you don't eat dairy foods, other sources include:

* Fortified soy milk and other fortified plant "milks"
* Fortified breakfast cereal
* Fortified orange juice
* Fish that contain small bones, such as sardines and canned salmon
* Almonds, hazelnuts, and Brazil nuts
* Sesame seeds and tahini
* Tofu and other soy products
* White or whole wheat bread made from calcium-fortified flour
* Legumes
* Green leafy vegetables
* Dried figs

Supernutrient: VITAMIN D

Importance: Vitamin D plays a pivotal role in the control of calcium absorption, and in bone growth. Researchers have recently found that low levels of vitamin D are more common than was previously thought, including among pregnant women.

Intake: Most of the vitamin D we require comes from the action of sunlight on our skin. During pregnancy and breast-feeding, an additional supplement of 10 mcg per day is recommended.

Where to find it: Foods generally contain little vitamin D, apart from fortified products. The best sources are:

* Fortified margarines and spreads
* Fortified products such as soy milks, yogurts, and breakfast cereals
* Oil-rich fish (but eat in limited amounts; see page 27)
* Meat
* Eggs
* Dairy products

Supernutrient: VITAMIN C

Importance: Vitamin C has a range of roles that are vital to an unborn baby's development, including

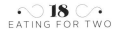

its function in the formation of skin and bone. Particular attention also needs to be paid to vitamin C because of its role in iron absorption.

Intake: The recommended intake of vitamin C increases during pregnancy. It's recommended that you try to include a source at each meal, both to meet your needs and to maximize iron absorption. People who smoke have been found to have lower vitamin C intake—this is particularly worrying because people who smoke actually require higher amounts of this vitamin.

Where to find it: Sources of vitamin C include:
* Berries and currants
* Citrus fruits
* Melon
* Kiwifruit
* Peppers, broccoli, cabbage, and kale
* Tomatoes

Note that foods must be eaten raw or very lightly cooked, otherwise vitamin C is destroyed.

Supernutrient: MAGNESIUM

Importance: Magnesium is the second-most abundant mineral in the body (so your baby needs to accumulate a lot of it), and its roles include skeletal development and energy metabolism. Research has suggested that women with lower magnesium levels may be at higher risk of premature labor as well as having babies with a lower birth weight.

Intake: Requirements increase during breast-feeding, though given the importance of this mineral to your baby during pregnancy, it's something to watch throughout pregnancy as well.

Where to find it: Rich sources of magnesium include:
* Green leafy vegetables
* Whole-grain cereal products
* Nuts
* Seeds

Supernutrient: ZINC

Importance: Zinc is required for cell division, for the formation of muscle, and for energy metabolism—thus it's critical to your baby's development. Scientists have reported a possible link between low zinc levels and premature birth and lower birth weight. While more research is required, it's worth ensuring a healthy zinc intake by regularly eating the foods listed below.

Intake: While the requirement for zinc doesn't increase during pregnancy, significantly more is required while breast-feeding.

Where to find it: Easily absorbed sources include:
* Red meat
* Fish and shellfish
* Poultry and eggs
* Dairy foods

Sources that are less easily absorbed include:
* Legumes
* Whole-grain foods
* Green leafy vegetables
* Nuts
* Wheat germ
* Pumpkin and sunflower seeds

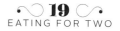

Should I buy organic foods?

This issue is tricky because there have been many studies comparing organic and nonorganic foods, with differing results. The UK's Food Standards Agency (FSA) has helped to clarify the situation by analyzing all the scientifically credible studies. They found that, overall, there were no significant nutritional differences between organic and nonorganic foods. The FSA also maintains strict control over additive and pesticide residue levels in the UK; organic and nonorganic foods must conform to the same guidelines for safe levels.

What this means is that you can feel free to buy organic if your budget allows, but don't be concerned that you are compromising your baby's nutrition or safety if you choose nonorganic. A much higher priority is making sure you include all the fruit, vegetables, and other foods that your body requires.

Do I need a supplement?

Apart from additional folic acid and vitamin D (see page 6), most women do not need a vitamin or mineral supplement while pregnant. Exceptions may be women who develop iron-deficiency anemia, those who don't or can't eat dairy foods or fish, and vegans or vegetarians who may also run low on certain nutrients. Because of the risks from vitamin A, only multivitamin and mineral supplements designed for pregnancy should be taken. Discuss taking any other supplements than these with your ob-gyn or pharmacist.

Playing it safe with food

Good food hygiene is critical during pregnancy. Pregnant women are more susceptible to some types of food poisoning, and the risks are more serious (see page 25). For that reason, I've included information on storing, preparing, and cooking food safely. This is probably information you're aware of already, but it's worth reviewing the guidelines because they're just so important at this time.

Storing foods

One basic principle of food safety is to keep hot food hot and cold food cold. This minimizes the time food spends in the "danger zone" temperatures, between 40°F and 145°F, when bacteria multiply at an alarming rate. Another is to prevent raw foods such as poultry from contaminating other foods or utensils. There are also strict guidelines on the length of time food can be safely stored.

❋ Monitor your refrigerator:
  • Make sure it is set at 40°F or below and working correctly. You can get a refrigerator thermometer to check this.
  • Store uncooked meat, fish, and poultry separately from cooked and ready-to-eat foods and those that will be eaten raw. Don't store uncooked meat, fish, or poultry above other foods in the fridge, to avoid possible contamination from drips.
  • Throw away foods if they are past their "use by" date.
  • Refrigerate leftover food promptly and throw it away after 24 hours if you haven't eaten it.

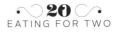

* Check food labels for storage instructions and follow them.
* Eat ready-to-eat foods and other perishable items as soon as possible after buying them.
* If food has been out of the fridge for two hours it should not be eaten.

Safe food preparation

One of the most important principles of safe food preparation is to prevent foods such as poultry from contaminating cooked foods or those that will be eaten raw. Another is to minimize bacteria on food and in cooking areas. Follow these guidelines to keep food safe:
* Wash your hands before and after handling food.
* Keep your kitchen surfaces, kitchen towels, and cooking utensils very clean.
* Keep pets away from food preparation areas and utensils.
* Wash utensils, cutting boards, surfaces, and your hands thoroughly after preparing uncooked foods, especially poultry, fish, and meat. Do not use the same area for preparing food to be eaten raw unless it and all equipment have been thoroughly cleaned.
* Wash raw fruit and vegetables thoroughly under running tap water before eating them.

Cooking food safely

It's particularly important during pregnancy that food is fully cooked—this kills bacteria such as *Listeria* (though some bacteria also produce toxins that are not destroyed by heating). Be sure to:
* Fully cook raw animal foods, such as meat, fish, and poultry.

* Heat prepared meals or reheated food until they're piping hot all the way through.
* Keep hot food hot until you are ready to eat it.
* Cook eggs until the yolk and white are hard, and avoid raw or undercooked eggs in foods such as soufflés, mousses, and homemade mayonnaise.

Staying active

Pregnancy has traditionally been seen as a time to sit down and put your feet up. However, if you are used to exercising, there's no need to give it up, though you will need to tone it down a bit as the pregnancy progresses. And even if you usually take it easy, a little light activity will help keep your body in shape. Thirty minutes of light activity is recommended each day during pregnancy (though you should start with up to three 15-minute sessions a week if you are not used to exercising). This has benefits both during and after the pregnancy, with the bonus that being fitter will help your body cope better with the marathon that is giving birth.

While you may be used to jogging 'til you drop, there are certain considerations to keep in mind while you're pregnant. Don't exercise too strenuously—you should be able to maintain a conversation while exercising without becoming breathless. Pregnancy alone can be very tiring, so avoid exercising to exhaustion. After 16 weeks you'll need to avoid exercises that involve lying on your back because of the pressure of the baby's weight on blood vessels, and always avoid contact sports or those with a risk of falling or being hit, such as cycling, skiing, and racquetball. Take extra care to acclimatize before being active if you are at high elevation, and take it easy in hot weather. Good activities to try during pregnancy include swimming and water aerobics (the water helps support your body), walking, and pregnancy yoga classes.

Remember to talk your exercise plans through with your ob-gyn if you have any health issues or are not used to exercising. Be sure to drink extra fluid when exercising, especially in hot weather, and always stop any activity that is causing discomfort.

I'm not pregnant yet. How can I prepare for pregnancy?

It's impossible to start following all the pregnancy guidelines as soon as you become pregnant, because it's always a few weeks before you find out. Thus it is wise to start taking the following precautions if you are trying to conceive:

❋ Start taking folic acid supplements: Take 400 mcg daily when trying to conceive and for the first three months of pregnancy. Some people need to take a higher dose (see page 6).

❋ Your chance of conceiving, your health, and that of your unborn baby can all be improved if you are a healthy weight. If you are over- or underweight, use the time before you get pregnant to lose or gain weight (by following a healthy diet), and aim to be within or closer to your optimal weight range (see page 9).

❋ Even if you don't need to gain or lose weight, following a nutritious diet before you become pregnant helps you build peak nutrient stores for pregnancy. This is particularly important for iron, as iron-deficiency anemia is a common problem during pregnancy.

❋ Early pregnancy is when your baby is beginning to develop and most vulnerable. If you start limiting alcohol and caffeinated drinks before you're pregnant, you'll be safeguarding your baby from the start.

❋ If you start paying extra attention to food hygiene now, you'll be in the habit when you get pregnant.

You'll find more information on all these points elsewhere in Eating for Two.

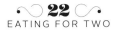

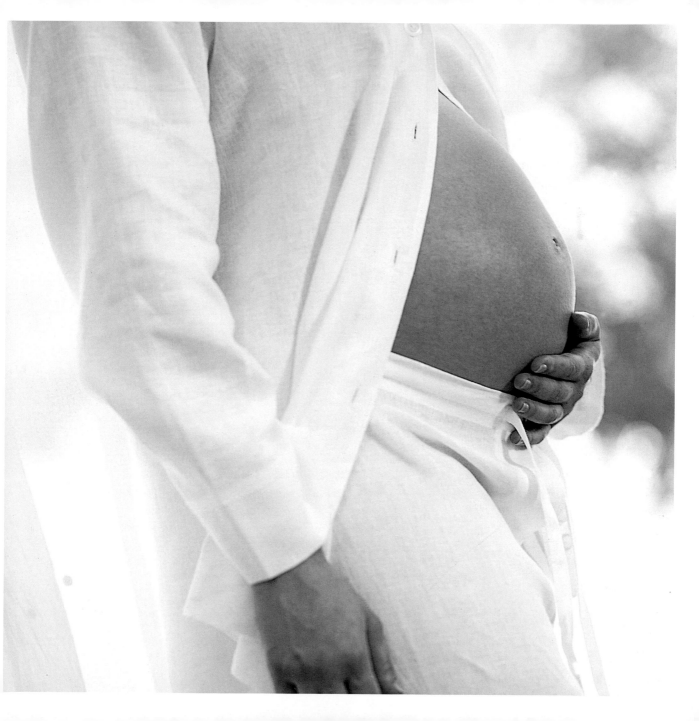

2: The First Trimester

The First Trimester: A critical time for nutrition
You're pregnant! You may not feel any different yet, but inside you is your tiny new child. Her cells are rapidly dividing and forming a multitude of different body parts, from brain to eyes to heart. It's not the only thing growing. Your baby will be nourished via the placenta, her link with the outside world, that is now forming inside you. Her home, your uterus, also begins to grow. All of these vital processes depend on nutrients, such as vitamins and minerals, supplied by your diet. This is happening at a time when it may become quite difficult to eat well. The first trimester is notorious for morning sickness, and can also be a time of food cravings. Read more about these conditions and how to handle them later in the chapter.

Nutrition priorities in the first trimester
You might think that all of this growth would require a lot of extra calories—actually the opposite is true (see Pregnancy Myth Buster box, opposite). However, it is a time to make sure the calories we do take in are of the best quality. That means focusing on healthy options from the core food groups because they offer the maximum amount of nutrients—vitamins, minerals, protein, and so on. It also means ditching the junk food that brings a lot of calories from fat and sugar, but few useful nutrients.

This early stage of pregnancy is particularly critical for your baby—it's the time when her development is most vulnerable, and this is affected by what you eat in two quite different ways. Nutrients are essential to ensure normal formation of your baby's physical structure and organs, including her brain. In addition, your baby is particularly sensitive to a range of harmful substances at this time. It's a time to be especially vigilant about guidelines about avoiding alcohol, maintaining food safety, and keeping clear of foods such as soft blue cheese (see page 28) or liver (see page 26), as these can occasionally cause problems during pregnancy.

Eating well in the first months of pregnancy can be challenging. As well as getting your head around all this new information, you may also be coping with morning sickness, extreme tiredness, and cravings. Morning sickness can lead to weight loss or, surprisingly, to weight gain due to the frequent snacking that can relieve nausea. Cravings can also tempt you with less nutritious foods. This is why choosing the right meals and snacks can be very important. Start with the information on food groups in chapter 1, and aim to eat about the same number of calories as you did before you became pregnant. Read on to find out what changes you may need to make to your usual choices to eat safely during pregnancy.

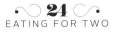

You and Your Baby: 0–3 months

You

The hormones that are flooding your body have myriad effects on your nutritional intake, from causing morning sickness to increasing the chance of indigestion and constipation.

• • •

Your body begins to make almost twice as much blood for the developing blood supply of the baby and placenta, so it's important to include plenty of iron-rich foods in your diet.

• • •

A healthy weight gain in this trimester is from about 1.1 to 4.4 pounds.

Your baby

The first trimester of your pregnancy is when the most rapid changes occur as your baby's organs are being formed.

• • •

By 12 weeks your baby is able to yawn, suck, swallow, and move her fingers.

• • •

By 12 weeks the baby is only about as long as your middle finger (3 inches) and weighs about 1.5 ounces.

What to eat and what to avoid

One of the most critical things to learn in early pregnancy is what foods to avoid. Some foods that are perfectly innocuous when you're not pregnant can cause major health issues for unborn babies, and it's essential that you are aware of them from as early as possible in the pregnancy. While the chance of any harm being caused is extremely slim, the consequences can be life-threatening for your baby. The two main areas of concern are various types of food poisoning, and substances in food that are potentially dangerous to unborn babies.

Pregnancy Myth Buster: Now that I'm pregnant, I can eat as much as I like!

Pregnancy is often seen as a time to forget diets, throw away the scales, and eat whatever you like. The combination of food cravings and knowing that weight gain is inevitable and even necessary can fuel temptation to eat fatty and sugary foods, with the excuse that you are "eating for two." In reality, while there are now two of you, your body is more efficient during pregnancy, and you don't need to eat extra calories for the first two trimesters. Even during the third trimester, only an extra 200 calories are needed each day, on average, and less if you were overweight at the beginning of pregnancy.

It can be tempting to throw caution to the wind, but this can mean gaining more weight than recommended. Excess weight gain can increase the risk of problems such as preeclampsia (see page 126) and diabetes during pregnancy, not to mention carrying extra weight after the birth that can be very difficult to lose. It can also be a result of choosing foods that are higher in fat and sugar, but possibly lower in the vitamins and minerals crucial to your baby's development. On the bright side, eating a nutritious diet that does supply all your baby's essential nutrients is unlikely to lead to excess weight, and is the best start in life for your baby.

Listeriosis

This is a type of food poisoning we don't hear much about, apart from during pregnancy. While it rarely causes problems for women who aren't pregnant, those who are pregnant are twenty times more likely to get sick from *Listeria* bacteria. It may cause only

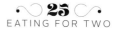

25
EATING FOR TWO

a flu-like illness in the mother, but can result in miscarriage or severe illness in an unborn baby.

The foods that are most likely to contain *Listeria* bacteria are certain cheeses, unpasteurized milk (from cows, sheep, and goats) and some foods made from unpasteurized milk, and ready-made cold foods that will be eaten cold. This includes foods such as pâté, prepared salads, pies, and quiches.

The area that causes most confusion is cheese. Many pregnant women know they need to avoid some cheese—but which ones? The more dangerous ones are mold-ripened and softer cheeses (it's easier for the bacteria to grow because of the higher water content in these cheeses). See the box on page 28 for more information about choosing cheese.

It's also recommended that pregnant women avoid eating any type of pâté, unpasteurized milk, and foods made from unpasteurized milk. In addition, pregnant women should avoid eating all deli meats and smoked seafood. You may choose to avoid these other foods too. Note that it particularly affects lunch, because it rules out many prepackaged sandwiches such as those made with ham, chicken, or smoked salmon.

Unlike most bacteria, *Listeria* can grow and multiply in some foods kept in the fridge—another reason why good food safety habits are so important. *Listeria* is killed by pasteurization and cooking, which is why pasteurized milk and other dairy products such as yogurts are generally safe. Be especially careful to follow the food hygiene guidelines in chapter 1 (see page 20) to help reduce the risk of *Listeria*.

Toxoplasmosis

This problem can be caused by food we eat, particularly raw or undercooked meat (including raw cured meats such as salami and Parma ham) and unpasteurized milk. For this reason, you should take extra care to choose pasteurized dairy foods, cook meat thoroughly, and prevent raw meat from contaminating other foods and surfaces. Another main cause is cat feces, so you need to be more vigilant if cats are around. This includes wearing disposable gloves when dealing with cat litter or when gardening.

Vitamin A

You're probably thinking that vitamin A is essential for you and your developing baby, not something to avoid. That's partially true. While it is essential during pregnancy, very high intakes of vitamin A are associated with an increased risk of birth defects. For this reason pregnant women should not take vitamin supplements containing vitamin A. Liver and foods made from liver, including fish liver oils, pâté, and liverwurst, can also be high in vitamin A and should be avoided at this time. You'll get all you need from a healthy diet, particularly from foods such as dairy products, carrots, eggs, and green leafy vegetables. If you do need a vitamin supplement, note that those designed specifically for pregnancy will not contain vitamin A.

Salmonella and other food poisoning

Food poisoning can strike us whether pregnant or not. However, it's best to be extra vigilant with food hygiene when pregnant, because some types such

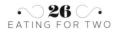

as salmonella and campylobacter can occasionally cause miscarriage or premature labor. Be especially careful to avoid eating undercooked or raw eggs (such as in homemade mayonnaise, mousses, and soufflés), and to cook poultry thoroughly.

Fish, including oil-rich fish

Yes, oil-rich fish are those that supply the healthy fish oils. They are a critical part of your diet during pregnancy, but the types of fish that contain these oils also contain small amounts of contaminants such as mercury and dioxins. Eating too much creates a risk of damage to your baby's nervous system. This means it's a balancing act between eating enough oil-rich fish for the healthy oils your developing baby needs, but not so much that there is a risk of any damage.

It's recommended that you:

❋ Limit your intake of oil-rich fish to no more than 2 portions a week. This includes fresh salmon, mackerel, herring, trout, sardines, and tuna, and the canned versions of all but the tuna.

❋ Avoid eating shark, swordfish, and marlin altogether.

❋ Limit the amount of tuna in your diet. Don't eat more than:

- 2 tuna steaks a week
  (about 5 ounces cooked or 6 ounces raw).
- 4 medium-sized cans of tuna a week
  (about 5 ounces when drained).

❋ Limit a number of other varieties of fish to no more than 2 portions a week. These are:

- Dogfish
- Sea bass
- Sea bream
- Turbot
- Halibut
- Crab

Raw fish and shellfish

Raw shellfish is another food that carries an increased risk of food poisoning—stick to cooked shellfish instead.

Raw fish can occasionally contain tiny worms that can make people sick. The worms are killed by freezing, smoking, or cooking the fish, so cooked fish should be safe to eat. Smoked fish such as smoked salmon will be safe with respect to the worms, but see the note on page 26 regarding deli meat and smoked fish.

Herbal medicines and supplements

Your pregnancy is a time to avoid taking any unnecessary medications, herbal medicines, or supplements, especially in the first trimester. If you haven't done so already, check with your ob-gyn or pharmacist about any prescribed or over-the-counter medications or supplements you are taking.

There is often little research on the safety of herbal medicines and supplements during pregnancy, so especially at this critical time it's better to be safe than sorry. This doesn't apply to herbs used in cooking, which are safe to use in normal amounts.

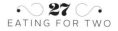

Allergy issues

Unless you yourself have a nut allergy, there's no need to avoid eating nuts or products containing them during your pregnancy. This may seem confusing because the advice has changed over the last few years—if this is your second pregnancy, you may find the advice is different. Scientists used to advise that women with a family history of allergies should avoid eating peanuts during pregnancy, but they found that there was no clear evidence that this would change the risk of allergies in their children. One factor they found did help to reduce allergy risk was to avoid smoking and exposure to secondhand smoke during the pregnancy.

A study has also found that mothers eating a diet higher in green and yellow vegetables and citrus fruits during pregnancy saw a lower incidence of eczema in their children. While more research is needed to confirm the association, there's certainly no harm and a lot of benefits in eating healthy amounts of these vegetables and citrus fruits.

Licorice

Scandinavian studies have found that eating large amounts of licorice during pregnancy could be linked to shorter pregnancies, and lower cognitive ability and behavioral problems in children. It's believed to be due to the licorice root (*Glycyrrhiza*) used to flavor the licorice. To be safe, I suggest you eat it in moderation. Some is flavored with anise oil, which is not linked to the problem.

Sprouts

Sprouts or sprouted seeds are occasionally linked to food poisoning outbreaks, so pregnant women should avoid eating them raw. Eat only sprouts that have been cooked through until piping hot.

Choosing cheese

When we are faced with the multitude of cheeses on the supermarket shelf, it can be hard to sort the safe options from the no-go varieties. Here's a guide to the more common types:

Enjoy these

✻ *Cheddar, Colby, Wensleydale, Emmental, gouda, Gruyère, Jarlsberg, and similar hard cheeses*
✻ *Cottage cheese, ricotta, Monterey Jack, and mozzarella made from pasteurized milk*
✻ *Parmesan*
✻ *Feta, paneer, and haloumi if made from pasteurized milk*
✻ *Cream cheese, processed cheese, and processed cheese spreads if made from pasteurized milk*
✻ *Hard blue cheese such as Stilton*
✻ *Cooked, hot versions of the cheeses to steer clear of, such as a hot goat cheese tart*

Steer clear of these

✻ *Brie or blue Brie*
✻ *Camembert*
✻ *Gorgonzola*
✻ *Danish blue*
✻ *Roquefort*
✻ *Other soft blue cheeses*
✻ *Soft, mold-ripened cheeses made from goat's or sheep's milk, such as chèvre*

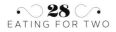

What to drink and what to avoid

Drinks during pregnancy range from those that we need more of to those that should be limited, to those that should be avoided. Here's some advice on what to fill your glass with for the next nine months:

Healthy hydration

It can be difficult staying hydrated when you're not pregnant, but it's even more important at the moment. During pregnancy, your fluid requirement increases a little: The American Institute of Medicine recommends an extra 8 ounces per day. This is largely because of the increase in the amount of fluid you are carrying in your body, including your blood and that of your baby, plus the amniotic fluid. As a rule, aim for 8 to 10 cups of fluid each day, and more during hot weather. See the box on page 30 for more information.

Alcohol

One benefit of morning sickness is that many women find they have no desire to drink alcohol at all during the first few months of pregnancy. This is just as well because the first trimester is the time when an unborn baby is most susceptible to alcohol passing through from the mother's bloodstream. For this reason, the UK's NHS and National Institute for Clinical Excellence (NICE) and the U.S. Surgeon General recommend that women abstain from drinking any alcohol during the first trimester. The UK's NHS and the U.S. Surgeon General also warn against drinking any alcohol during the rest of the pregnancy, because the alcohol passes through the placenta to the baby, whose developing liver cannot process alcohol as an adult liver can. It's thought this can lead to developmental problems, with binge drinking being particularly harmful.

Caffeine

While there's no problem with moderate amounts of caffeine during pregnancy, higher amounts have been linked to an increased risk of miscarriage and lower birth weights. Pregnant women should therefore limit caffeine intake to 200 mg per day.

To translate this into caffeine amounts in your everyday drinks and food:

✳ A single espresso shot contains about 75 mg of caffeine. "Small"-size coffee shop drinks such as cappuccinos or lattes tend to be made with one espresso shot, so they will also contain about 75 mg of caffeine. Remember that larger coffees tend to be made with two or even three shots of espresso, so check with the person making the coffee and multiply the 75 mg accordingly.

✳ A mug of instant coffee contains 100 mg.

✳ Filter coffee is higher at 140 mg caffeine in a mug. Remember that many coffee shop measures are bigger than this.

✳ A mug of tea contains 75 mg.

✳ A can of cola contains 40 mg.

✳ A can of energy contains 80 mg.

✳ A milk chocolate bar (50 g/2 oz) contains 25 mg.

✳ A dark chocolate bar (50 g/2 oz) contains 50 mg.

So you could still have your small daily latte, a cup of tea, and a few squares of chocolate as an after-dinner treat and stay well within the limit. Be aware that some medications, particularly those for colds,

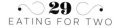

flu, and headaches, also contain caffeine, and there are small amounts in other coffee- or chocolate-flavored foods such as desserts.

It can be difficult to cut down on tea and coffee when they are a regular part of your day. Try swapping them for decaf versions, or drink more juices or sparkling mineral water with a refreshing slice of lemon. Make sure you allow time for enough sleep to be sure you aren't depending on caffeine to keep you alert. And remember that occasionally going a little over the 200 mg limit is unlikely to cause harm to your baby—it's what you do most of the time that counts.

Herbal teas

Some women feel herbal teas are beneficial during pregnancy, but, to be safe, you should speak to your health care professional before using them because many substances pass through the placenta and the developing baby is therefore being exposed. There are also some substances that are known not to be safe at times during pregnancy. For example, red raspberry leaf tea stimulates uterine contractions and should not be used early in the pregnancy.

For more on red raspberry leaf tea, which is often taken late in pregnancy, see the information in chapter 4 (page 126).

Special considerations if you are vegetarian or vegan

There's no reason why vegetarian or vegan moms-to-be should not follow a well-planned diet. These diets can make it more difficult to eat enough of certain nutrients, however, meaning extra thought and sometimes extra supplements may be required during pregnancy. Nutrients to think about include vitamin B_{12}, vitamin D, iron, and omega-3 oils, and for vegans also calcium, iodine, and riboflavin (vitamin B_2). See Pregnancy Supernutrients on page 16 for more on vegetarian sources of vitamin D, iron, calcium, and omega-3 oils.

Protein is found in many foods other than meat: Dairy foods, eggs, nuts, seeds, mycoprotein, and legumes (including soy-based foods such as tofu) are among the most valuable sources. If you eat eggs and dairy foods, you'll be likely to include plenty of animal-based protein; however, if you are vegan, it's essential that you take extra care to include a variety of plant-based protein sources each day. Again, there's more information on protein in chapter 1 (see page 10).

Pregnancy Myth Buster: We need to drink eight glasses of water a day

It's a common belief that we need to drink eight glasses of water a day (or a little more during pregnancy), and many people find that really difficult on top of the tea, juice, or other drinks we already enjoy. There's no need for this concern—all nonalcoholic drinks count toward the daily total. Of course, being pregnant, you will be avoiding alcohol and limiting caffeinated drinks. However, your 8 to 10 glasses of fluid a day could be made up of one glass of juice, a coffee and a tea, two glasses of flavored water, and four glasses of water, for example.

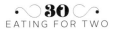

The main sources of vitamin B_2, vitamin B_{12}, and iodine are animal foods, so it's vital during pregnancy to be aware of the few vegetarian sources.

✻ Vitamin B_2: Dairy foods, eggs, and meat are a good source of vitamin B_2, also known as riboflavin, however, people who don't eat these foods will need to look to yeast extract, fortified breakfast cereals, fortified soy milk, green leafy vegetables, almonds, and soy beans.

✻ Vitamin B_{12}: This vitamin is found in all animal-based foods, but does not occur naturally in plant foods. Thus, if you are vegan, you will need to eat foods fortified with vitamin B_{12}, including fortified yeast extract, fortified soy or rice milk, fortified breakfast cereal, and fortified TVP.

✻ Iodine: Milk, fish, and shellfish are major sources of iodine. If you do not consume dairy products, sources of iodine include seaweed, iodized salt, and kelp-fortified yeast extracts.

You might wish to take a pregnancy multivitamin and mineral supplement if you are concerned about your intake of any vitamins and minerals, particularly if you are vegan. As for all pregnant women, a folic acid supplement is recommended for the first trimester of pregnancy (and before, if possible), and a vitamin D supplement throughout the pregnancy.

It can be very difficult to obtain omega-3 oils (the type found in oil-rich fish) from a vegetarian or vegan diet. This is because there are limited sources apart from fish. See the information on these oils on pages 12 and 13. Note that there are omega-3 supplements available that are made from microalgae, and therefore suitable if you are vegan.

Healthy habits

Pregnancy is the perfect time for a diet makeover, not just for while you are pregnant but to take on into breast-feeding and when the time comes to set a healthy example for your young child. Part of this involves adopting positive habits that promote healthy eating and also help maintain energy levels through the day. You could even start by writing down what you eat, and when, for a few days. Look through the results and see if there are any changes you could make. Here are a few areas to consider:

✻ Food groups: Look through the food group information in chapter 1. Are you eating what your body needs?

✻ Ditch the junk: Check how often you are eating fatty or sugary foods. Could some of these be replaced with more nutritious options?

✻ Start the day with breakfast: Breakfast is the meal we skip most often, and this is even more unwise during pregnancy. Studies show that people who eat breakfast tend to eat more nutritious diets overall, and pregnancy is the most important time for that. The same applies to skipping other meals—a constant supply of nutrients is critical.

✻ Healthy snacks: We often think of snacks as being less nutritious or less valuable than foods we eat at mealtimes; however, this is not the case. By choosing wisely from the food groups, and avoiding fatty and sugary foods, snacks can be a useful part of our diet.

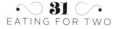

Top 10: Healthy handbag snacks
* ✽ Cereal bar
* ✽ Fruit-and-nut or seed bar
* ✽ Oatcakes (plain or flavored)
* ✽ Apple or any other non-squashable fruit
* ✽ Dried fruit
* ✽ Nuts (try almonds, peanuts, Brazil nuts, or walnuts)
* ✽ Whole-grain rice cakes (look for lower-salt types)
* ✽ Mixed seeds such as pumpkin and sunflower seeds (try the flavored varieties)
* ✽ Whole-grain crackers filled with peanut butter and jam
* ✽ Make up your own gourmet trail mix of raisins, dried cranberries, seeds, and nuts

Nutritional issues

Morning sickness

While not everyone suffers from morning sickness, nausea does affect most pregnant women and about half experience vomiting as well. The good news is that morning sickness generally subsides after the first trimester, though if you are the person affected, that may seem like an eternity. While few medications are available to help, certain eating habits can make a huge difference. Food may be the last thing you want to see when feeling nauseated, but eating small amounts regularly is key—an empty stomach makes the nausea worse in most people. And, of course, you still need to be taking in the nutrients your growing baby needs.

Try to avoid the temptation to live on crackers and cookies. They are a convenient snack but are not rich in the nutrients necessary for pregnancy.

Try dried fruit and nuts, a small bowl of breakfast cereal, or whole-grain crackers and cheese instead.

There is some evidence that ginger and possibly vitamin B_6 may help to reduce nausea—be sure to discuss this with your ob-gyn or pharmacist before taking any supplements, to make sure the level is safe.

See your ob-gyn if you are not managing to keep any food or fluids down. You may have a condition called hyperemesis gravidarum, which is vomiting severe enough to put you at risk of becoming very dehydrated. It is rare, but may require hospital treatment to give fluids via a drip.

Top 10 ways to beat morning sickness
* ✽ Start the day with a light snack before you actually get out of bed. You could keep a box of crackers by the bed, or maybe your partner will be thoughtful enough to bring you tea and dry toast.
* ✽ Eat a small, high-carbohydrate snack every hour or so.
* ✽ Minimize cooking smells by opening windows and using exhaust fans when cooking (easier said than done if it is winter). Eat in a different room from where food is prepared. Choose cool or cold foods, as these have less of an odor.
* ✽ Some people find that foods or drinks containing ginger help to relieve nausea. You could try ginger beer (nonalcoholic, of course), ginger ale, ginger cookies, or a stir-fry flavored with ginger.
* ✽ Avoid eating greasy foods because they'll sit in your stomach longer. Some women also feel better if they avoid eating spicy foods.

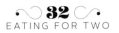

* Make meals that are quick to prepare—or try to get someone else to do it.
* Suck on a slice of lemon or a sour candy.
* Have a sip of a carbonated drink every few minutes when feeling nauseated.
* Eat smaller meals but include more snacks to compensate. Eat more at the times of day when you feel better.
* Don't drink much with meals (but compensate by sipping drinks regularly between meals). This will help prevent you from feeling as full at meals and help with nausea.

Food cravings and aversions

People always laugh about pregnant women craving crazy foods. While most cravings are not so amusing, they are very real. From chocolate to pickled onions, when they strike, they can be hard to resist. So long as you keep your overall diet balanced, there's no great risk of harm; in fact, aversions to alcohol and caffeine in early pregnancy may even be helpful. However, giving in to frequent cravings for potato chips or chocolate can mean filling up on junk food, with less space left for more nutritious fare.

If you plan ahead, you can turn your cravings into something healthy. For example, if you are craving crunchy chips, have a healthier option on hand such as crunchy cereal bars, carrot and celery sticks, or breadsticks. This way you'll get some vitamins, minerals, and fiber with every crunchy bite. If it's a sweet treat you're after, try strawberries, dried mango, a jam sandwich, or a fruit smoothie.

Cravings refer to a desire for foods, but occasionally pregnant women have an overwhelming appetite for substances that are not food, such as soil, match heads, or soap powder. This is a condition called pica, and unlike food cravings, it can be harmful if people eat what they crave. If you have cravings for nonfoods such as these, and you fear you may not be able to resist them, speak to your ob-gyn.

Fatigue

There's nothing quite as sapping as the tiredness that can descend during pregnancy. For many of us this is an unavoidable part of being pregnant; however, sometimes it can be due to iron-deficiency anemia. You will be given a blood test to check for this. Getting enough rest is also crucial. Another positive step you can take is to make sure your diet is optimal. This will help to keep energy levels as even as possible.

Review the guidelines for the food groups in chapter 1 (see page 13) to make sure you're eating all you require. Then be sure you're eating every few hours. Regular meals and snacks are key to keeping your body fueled—try to include some carbohydrates from grain foods or potatoes, and fruit or dairy foods (milk drinks, yogurt, or cottage cheese). Check out the glycemic index (GI) guidelines in the next chapter (see page 71) for carbs that may keep you filled and fueled for longer. Now, if you can just find a few minutes to put your feet up . . .

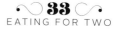

Pregnancy Myth Buster: I need to eat perfectly while I'm pregnant

There are many stresses during pregnancy, and food is a common one. Everyone wants to follow every guideline perfectly, but real life can get in the way. You may forget to take healthy snacks to work and have to rely on the snack machine. You may be stuck on a highway with no options apart from fast food. Or you may just have a really tough day and be desperate for a slice of rich chocolate cake. Please be reassured that as long as you are usually eating a balanced diet and taking the recommended vitamin supplements, your body will be receiving all the nutrients you need. The occasional slipup is no problem and is one thing you don't need to feel stressed about.

Breakfasts

8 tablespoons (1 stick) butter
1 cup (firmly packed) light
   brown sugar
⅔ cup whole wheat flour
1 cup all-purpose flour
1 teaspoon baking soda
½ teaspoon ground
   cinnamon
Large pinch of salt
½ cup chopped pecans
⅓ cup raisins
½ cup plain whole milk
   yogurt
1 teaspoon vanilla extract
2 large eggs
2 very ripe large bananas,
   mashed

Banana bread

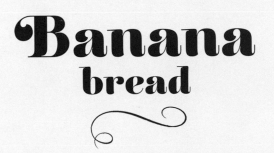

✳ Preheat the oven to 350°F. Line a 2-pound loaf pan (about 9 × 5 × 3½ inches) with parchment paper, with the parchment coming up the sides of the pan.

✳ Put the butter and sugar in a small saucepan. Heat until the butter has just melted, then set aside to cool slightly.

✳ In a large bowl, stir together the flours, baking soda, cinnamon, salt, pecans, and raisins. Whisk the yogurt, vanilla, and eggs into the melted butter, then add to the dry ingredients along with the bananas. Stir together and pour the mixture into the prepared pan.

✳ Bake for 1 hour to 1 hour 10 minutes, until risen and firm to the touch and a toothpick inserted in the center comes out clean. Let cool in the pan for 15 minutes, then transfer to a wire rack to cool completely. Store in an airtight container. Try spreading with low-fat cream cheese or drizzling with a little honey.

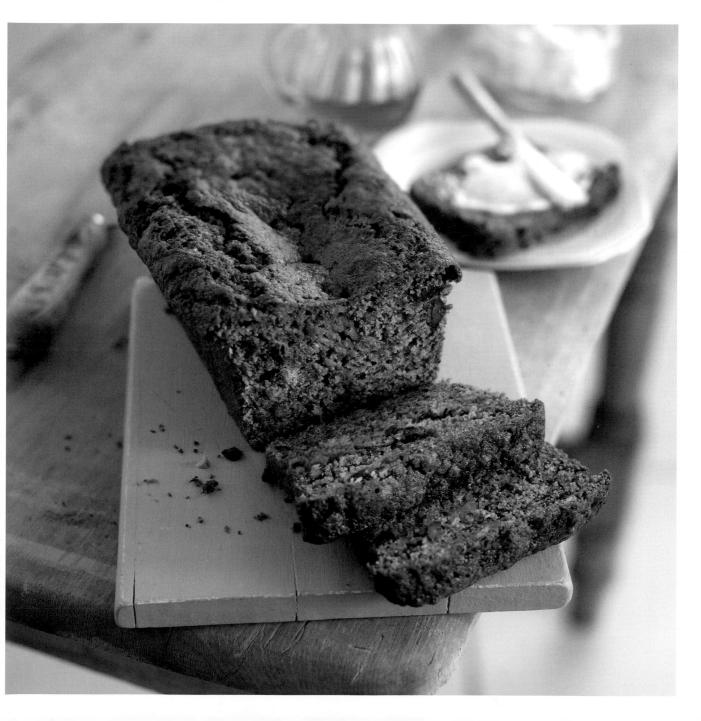

2½ cups quick-cooking oats
⅓ cup unsweetened
    shredded coconut
½ teaspoon ground
    cinnamon
¼ cup (firmly packed) light
    brown sugar
Large pinch of salt
2 tablespoons canola oil,
    plus extra for greasing
¼ cup honey
½ cup sliced almonds
    (you can vary the nuts,
    e.g., chopped pecans,
    walnuts, hazelnuts)
⅓ cup dried cranberries
½ cup dried apricots, cut
    into raisin-size pieces

Cinnamon almond granola

✶ ENERGY BOOST ✶

✶ Preheat the oven to 300°F. Lightly grease a large baking sheet.

✶ Put the oats, coconut, cinnamon, sugar, and salt in a large bowl and stir together. Drizzle with the oil and honey and stir until everything is thoroughly combined. Stir in the almonds. Spread the mixture out on the prepared baking sheet and bake for 20 minutes. Stir, and bake for 20 minutes more. Stir again, and bake for 5 to 10 minutes, until lightly toasted.

✶ Transfer the granola to a large bowl and let cool. Stir in the cranberries and apricots and store in an airtight container.

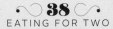

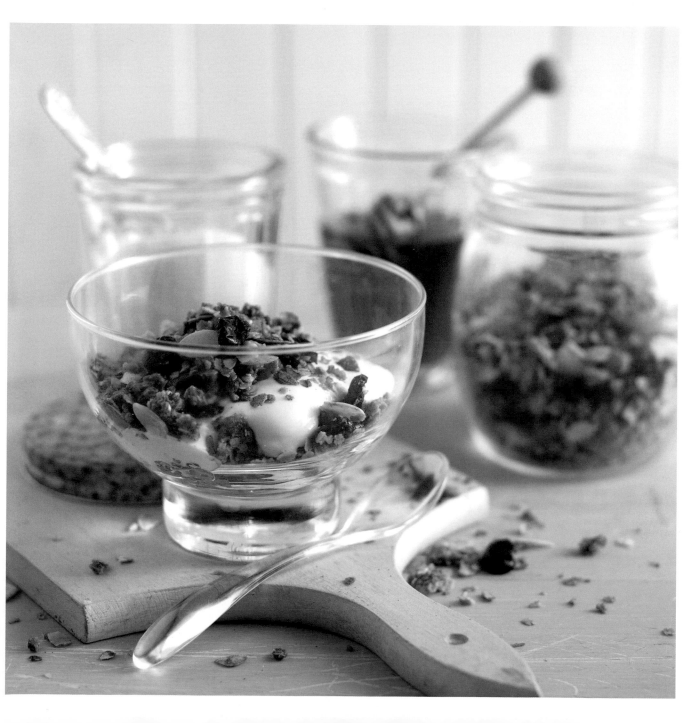

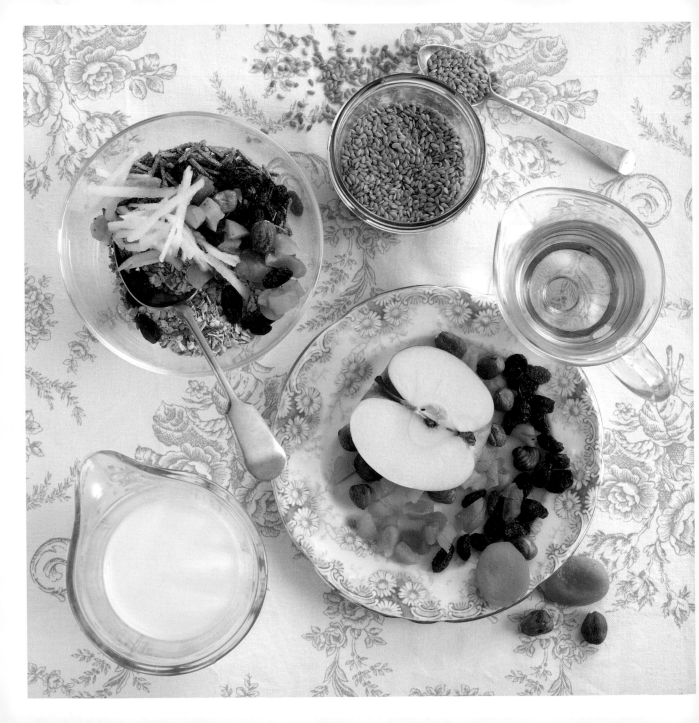

Oats, bran, and apple are all low-GI foods, meaning this is a great way to fuel your body through a busy morning. The flaxseed adds a boost of non-fish omega-3 oils, as well as valuable fiber.

• • •

MAKES 2 PORTIONS

½ cup quick-cooking oats

¾ cup All-Bran cereal

2 tablespoons golden flaxseed

2 tablespoons golden raisins

2 tablespoons chopped dried apricots

2 tablespoons coarsely chopped hazelnuts

½ cup apple juice

⅔ cup whole milk, plus extra (optional) for serving

½ apple, peeled and grated

Apple and hazelnut bircher muesli

✱ **FIBER-RICH FUEL** ✱

✱ Measure all of the ingredients into a mixing bowl. Stir together, then refrigerate for 15 minutes before serving with extra milk, if using.

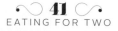

2 tablespoons butter

2 cups thinly sliced cremini mushrooms

2 to 3 drops Worcestershire sauce

¼ teaspoon Dijon mustard

3 tablespoons crème fraîche or sour cream (low-fat is fine)

1 English muffin, split and toasted

1 teaspoon chopped fresh parsley (optional)

Deviled
mushrooms

✴ Melt 1 tablespoon of the butter in a medium frying pan. Add the mushrooms and sauté over high heat for 6 to 8 minutes, until they are golden. Stir in the Worcestershire sauce and mustard. Remove from the heat and stir in the crème fraîche. Set the muffin halves, toasted side up, on a plate, spread with the remaining 1 tablespoon butter, and spoon on the mushrooms. Sprinkle with a little chopped parsley, if using.

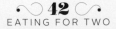

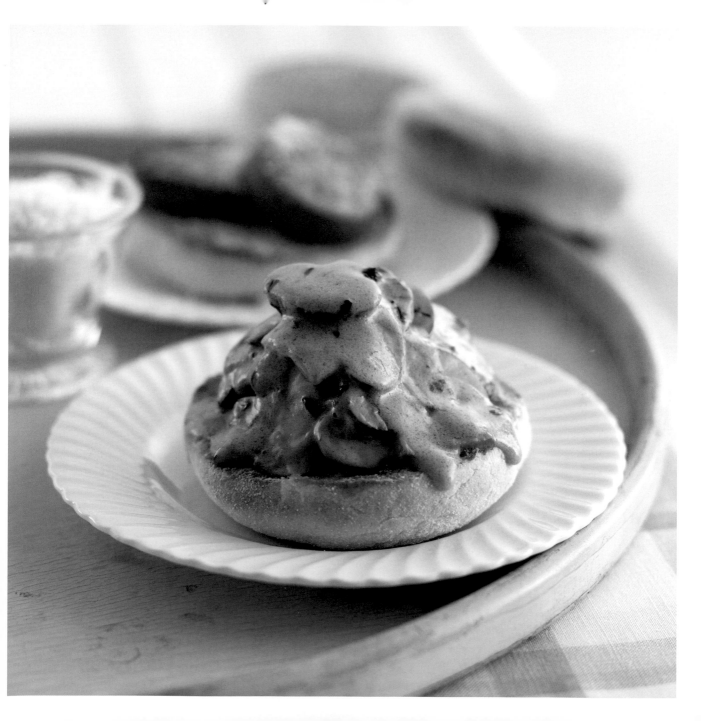

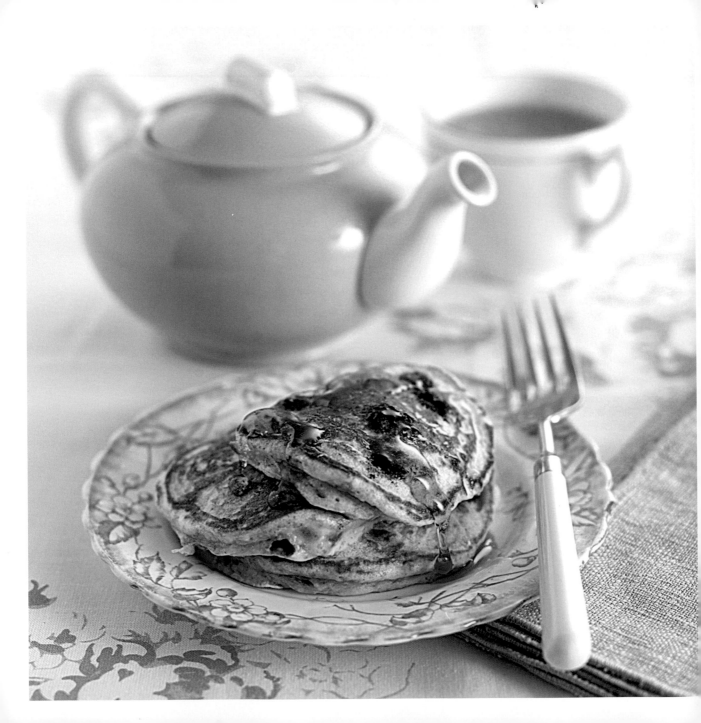

This mix is wonderful to have on hand so that you can whip up a batch of pancakes quickly. Rolled oats and whole wheat flour provide a fiber boost and mean that these will keep your body on the go for longer than regular pancakes.

• • •

MAKES ABOUT 2¾ CUPS MIX

1 cup quick-cooking oats
⅔ cup whole wheat flour
1 cup all-purpose flour
¼ cup superfine sugar
2 teaspoons baking powder
1 teaspoon baking soda
¼ teaspoon salt

MAKES 12 SMALL OR 8 LARGE PANCAKES

Multigrain pancakes

✶ Put all the ingredients in a food processor and whiz for 1 to 2 minutes, until the oats are finely ground. Transfer to an airtight container and store in a cool, dry place.

Plain pancakes

✶ To ¾ cup of the mix, add 1 egg and 6 tablespoons of milk. Mix and let stand for 3 to 5 minutes (the mixture will bubble slightly) as you preheat a large, heavy-bottomed frying pan. Drop the mixture into the pan (2 tablespoons per pancake for small, 3 tablespoons for large) and cook over medium-low heat until the undersides are golden, bubbles have appeared on the surface of the pancakes, and the surface is no longer runny. Flip the pancakes and cook for 1 minute, then transfer to plates. You may need to cook in batches. *More variations on page 46.*

Blueberry buttermilk

✴ Stir ¾ cup fresh blueberries into ¾ cup of the pancake mix. Add 6 tablespoons of buttermilk and 1 egg. Cook as on page 45.

Apple and raisin

✴ Stir ⅓ cup raisins and half a peeled and grated apple into ¾ cup of the pancake mix. Add ¼ cup of milk and 1 egg. Cook as on page 45.

With four types of fruit or juice, this smoothie packs a vitamin punch. Enjoy!

• • •

MAKES 2 GLASSES

2 ripe small bananas, sliced
1⅓ cups halved strawberries
¾ cups raspberries
¼ cup apple juice

Red fruit breakfast smoothie

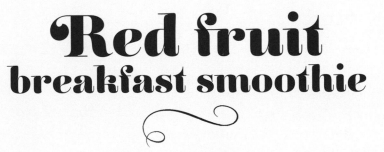

✴ HIGH IN VITAMIN C ✴

✴ Whiz the fruits and apple juice in a blender until smooth. Pass through a strainer into a pitcher. Refrigerate for 30 minutes before serving or pour into glasses and add some ice cubes.

2 medium tomatoes, sliced
1 tablespoon softened butter
½ small clove garlic,
    crushed
Salt and pepper
1 English muffin, split and
    toasted
1 tablespoon grated
    (or 6 shavings)
    Parmesan cheese

Grilled tomato and cheese

✳ Preheat the broiler. Place the tomatoes on a baking sheet. Broil for 2 to 4 minutes, until the slices start to wrinkle. Mix half the butter with the garlic and salt and pepper. Turn the tomatoes over and spread with the butter. Broil for 4 to 6 minutes more, until golden on top and cooked through. Spread the muffin with the remaining butter and set a few tomato slices on each muffin half. Top with the Parmesan.

1 tablespoon butter
1 tomato, seeded and diced
1 scallion, thinly sliced
2 eggs, beaten
1 tablespoon heavy cream
1 flour tortilla
¼ cup grated Cheddar
    cheese

Quick breakfast burrito

✳ Melt the butter and sauté the tomato and sliced scallion for a couple of minutes. Add the eggs and cook over medium-low heat until scrambled. Pour in the cream, cook for a few seconds, and remove from the heat. Warm the tortilla in the microwave or a dry frying pan. Spoon the scrambled egg mixture down the center and top with the grated Cheddar. Roll up.

1 tablespoon canola or olive oil
1 small red onion, thinly sliced
½ red bell pepper, seeded and
    thinly sliced
1 teaspoon balsamic vinegar
Large pinch of smoked Spanish
    paprika or pinch of ground
    coriander
2 tablespoons butter
3 eggs, beaten
1 tablespoon chopped fresh
    cilantro (optional)
Salt and pepper
2 large flour tortillas
3 tablespoons of your favorite
    store-bought salsa
Sour cream to serve (optional)

Breakfast burrito

✳ Heat the oil and sauté the onion and bell pepper for 5 minutes, or until soft. Add the balsamic vinegar and smoked paprika or ground coriander and cook for 1 minute. Set aside to cool slightly while you scramble the eggs.

✳ Melt the butter in a saucepan and add the eggs. Cook, stirring, until softly scrambled. Stir in the cilantro, if using, and season to taste with salt and pepper. Warm the tortillas in the microwave for about 10 seconds or in a dry frying pan for about 30 seconds.

✳ Divide the onion and pepper mixture between the tortillas, keeping it in the center. Add the eggs, then a spoonful of the salsa. Fold the edges in, then roll up the tortilla to make a burrito. Serve with a little sour cream, if using.

Tip:

The bell pepper and onion mixture can be made ahead. Cover and refrigerate until needed. Warm the pepper mixture in a saucepan, or in the microwave for 15 to 20 seconds.

Chicken

Porcini mushrooms are the kings of the mushroom family. They have a nutty, meaty flavor and a smooth, creamy texture. Dried porcini, widely available in supermarkets, add a delicious flavor to this dish. Soak in boiling water until they are reconstituted.

• • •

Chicken with wild mushroom and red pepper sauce

MAKES 2 PORTIONS
SUITABLE FOR FREEZING

Handful (about 2 tablespoons) of dried porcini mushrooms
⅔ cup boiling water
1 red bell pepper, seeded and sliced in half
2 tablespoons canola oil
2 skinless, boneless chicken breasts, sliced into thick strips
1 onion, chopped
2 cloves garlic, crushed
6 ounces mixed wild mushrooms, trimmed
⅔ cup chicken broth
Scant 1 cup heavy cream
1 teaspoon Worcestershire sauce
1 teaspoon lemon juice
2 teaspoons chopped fresh tarragon
Salt and pepper

✳ Put the porcini mushrooms in a bowl and add the boiling water. Let soak for 20 minutes. Lift the porcini out of the bowl, reserving the soaking liquid. Chop the porcini.

✳ Preheat the oven to 425°F. Put the bell pepper halves, cut side down, on a baking sheet. Roast for 20 to 25 minutes, until the skins are light brown. Remove from the oven, place in a bowl, and cover with plastic wrap. Once cool, remove the skin and slice the flesh into strips.

✳ Heat 1 tablespoon of the oil in a frying pan. Sauté the chicken until brown, then transfer to a plate. Add the remaining 1 tablespoon oil to the pan, then add the onion and garlic and sauté for 5 minutes. Add the chopped porcini and the wild mushrooms and sauté for 2 minutes. Strain the reserved porcini liquid and add to the pan with the broth, bring to a boil, then let it bubble until reduced by half. Add the heavy cream and the chicken and simmer for 2 minutes. Add the Worcestershire sauce, lemon juice, and tarragon and cook for another 2 to 3 minutes, until the chicken has cooked through. Season to taste with salt and pepper, then stir in the bell pepper and serve.

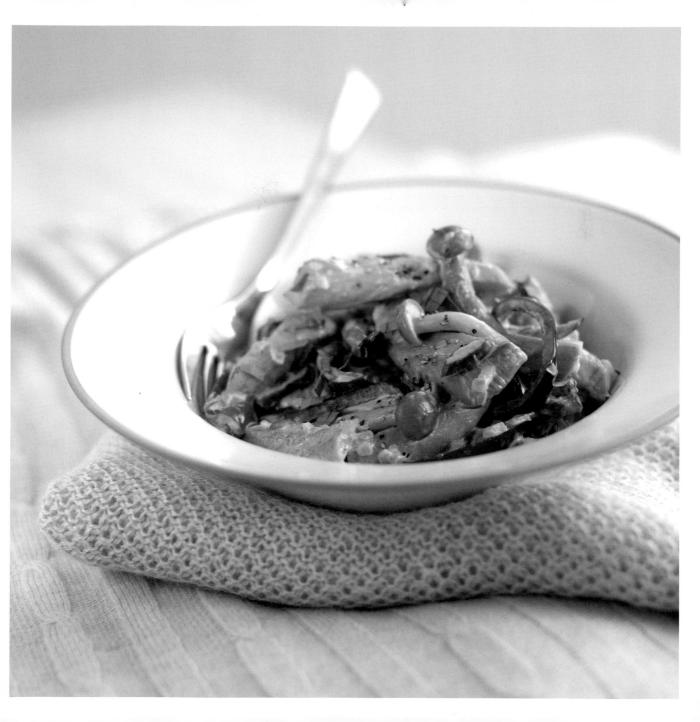

8 ounces fusilli pasta

5 tablespoons butter

2 cups thinly sliced cremini mushrooms

1 shallot, thinly sliced

⅓ cup all-purpose flour

1 tablespoon white wine vinegar

1⅔ cups milk

1⅔ cups chicken broth

3 cups (loosely packed) shredded cooked chicken (2 breasts)

¼ cup heavy cream (optional)

Salt and pepper

¼ cup grated Gruyère cheese

¼ cup grated Cheddar cheese

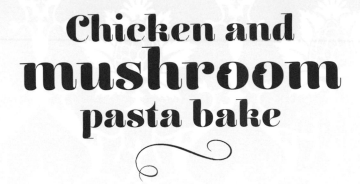

Chicken and mushroom pasta bake

✳ Cook the pasta for 1 minute less than the time stated on the package. Drain and set aside.

✳ Melt 2 tablespoons of the butter in a large saucepan and sauté the mushrooms until golden brown. Transfer to a plate and set aside.

✳ Melt the remaining 3 tablespoons butter in a saucepan and sauté the shallot for 2 to 3 minutes, until soft. Stir in the flour to make a paste, then add the vinegar and cook for 1 minute. Stir in the milk, a little at a time, to make a smooth sauce, then stir in the broth. Cook the sauce, stirring constantly, until it thickens very slightly and comes to a boil. Remove from the heat and stir in the chicken, mushrooms, pasta, and cream, if using. Season to taste with salt and pepper.

✳ Transfer to one large or two smaller baking dishes and sprinkle with the Gruyère and Cheddar. Heat through in the oven at 350°F for about 15 minutes and then finish off under a preheated broiler until golden.

This is a good dish to squirrel away in the freezer so that you have some delicious food ready to heat once you've had your baby.

• • •

MAKES 3 PORTIONS
SUITABLE FOR FREEZING

3 tablespoons canola oil
1 onion, coarsely chopped
1 cup grated carrot
½-inch piece fresh ginger, peeled and grated
2 cloves garlic, crushed
2 teaspoons mild korma curry paste (such as Patak's)
2 teaspoons ground cumin
1½ teaspoons ground cinnamon
1 teaspoon ground turmeric
3 dried apricots, coarsely chopped
One 14-ounce can diced tomatoes
1⅔ cups water
2 teaspoons chicken bouillon powder
1 to 2 teaspoons honey
2 teaspoons lemon juice
12 ounces skinless, boneless chicken breast, cut into 1½-inch pieces
1 teaspoon paprika
Salt and pepper
¾ cup cubed eggplant
½ cup peeled and cubed sweet potato

Chicken
tagine

✳ First make the tagine sauce: Heat 2 tablespoons of the oil in a deep saucepan. Add the onion, carrot, ginger, and garlic. Sauté for 10 minutes, or until softened. Add the curry paste, cumin, cinnamon, ½ teaspoon of the turmeric, and the apricots. Cook for 2 minutes, then add the tomatoes, water, bouillon powder, honey, and lemon juice. Simmer, covered, for 10 minutes.

✳ Meanwhile, toss the chicken pieces with the paprika and the remaining ½ teaspoon turmeric and season with salt and pepper. Heat the remaining 1 tablespoon oil in a frying pan. Brown the chicken until golden. Add the eggplant and sweet potato to the sauce and simmer for 5 minutes, then add the chicken and continue to cook for another 5 minutes, or until tender and cooked through. Serve with couscous or rice.

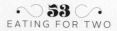

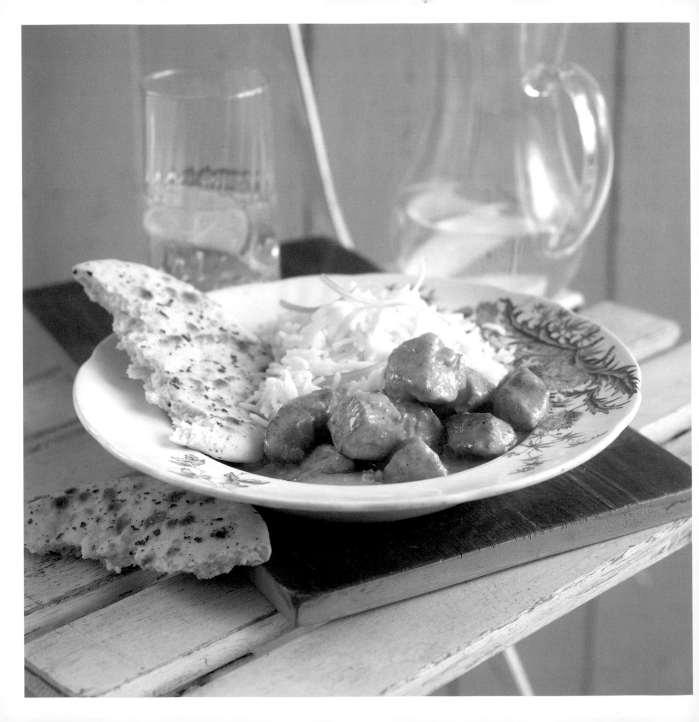

Eating curry is often suggested as a means of bringing on labor, but I'm not sure there's any scientific evidence to back it up. To be safe you may not want to order a hot vindaloo, but this mild, creamy korma is quick to make and bursting with flavor.

• • •

MAKES 2 OR 3 PORTIONS
SUITABLE FOR FREEZING

2 tablespoons canola oil
2 skinless, boneless chicken breasts, cut into bite-size pieces
1 large onion, coarsely chopped
1 red chile, seeded and diced
2 cloves garlic, crushed
½ teaspoon ground ginger
3 tablespoons mild korma curry paste (such as Patak's)
One 13.5-ounce can coconut milk
⅔ cup chicken broth
2 teaspoons mango chutney
2 tablespoons heavy cream
Salt and pepper
2 scallions, sliced (optional)

Quick creamy chicken curry

✶ Heat 1 tablespoon of the oil in a deep frying pan or wok. Sauté the chicken until brown, then transfer to a plate and set aside. Heat the remaining 1 tablespoon oil. Add the onion, chile, and garlic.

✶ Sauté for 5 minutes, or until nearly softened. Add the ginger and curry paste. Blend in the coconut milk and broth. Bring to a boil and reduce until the sauce has thickened. Add the mango chutney, cream, and chicken. Simmer for 5 minutes, or until the chicken is cooked through. Season well with salt and pepper. Serve with rice and/or naan bread and garnish with scallions, if using.

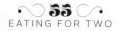

Noodles are a low-GI food, which means the carbohydrate is absorbed more slowly, and may keep you fuller for longer.

• • •

MAKES 3 PORTIONS

3 tablespoons mirin
5 tablespoons soy sauce
3 tablespoons honey
2 teaspoons rice vinegar
1 teaspoon grated fresh ginger
1 clove garlic, crushed
4 skinless, boneless chicken thighs, cut into large chunks
Salt and pepper
3 tablespoons canola oil
4 ounces medium (chow mein) egg noodles
2 scallions, thinly sliced
1 red onion, sliced
1 large zucchini, sliced into batons
1 large carrot, sliced into batons
1 cup thinly sliced cremini mushrooms
5 tablespoons chicken broth or water
4 teaspoons sweet chili sauce

Yakitori chicken kebabs with noodles

✳ Preheat the oven to 425°F.

✳ Measure the mirin, 3 tablespoons of the soy sauce, the honey, vinegar, ginger, and garlic into a small saucepan. Bring to a boil, then reduce by a third, stirring. Let cool.

✳ Add the chicken and refrigerate for 30 minutes. Drain, season with salt and pepper, and thread onto 6 skewers. Heat 2 tablespoons of the oil in a frying pan. Brown the skewers for 1 to 2 minutes on each side, until the chicken is golden, then place on a baking sheet. Bake for 12 to 15 minutes, until the chicken is cooked through.

✳ Meanwhile, cook the noodles in boiling salted water, following the package instructions. Drain.

✳ Heat the remaining 1 tablespoon oil in a frying pan or wok. Cook the scallions and onion for 5 minutes, then add the rest of the vegetables and cook for 2 to 3 minutes more. Add the noodles, broth, chili sauce, the remaining 2 tablespoons soy sauce, and salt and pepper to taste. Serve with the kebabs.

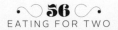

This delicious recipe is very simple to prepare and helps to maximize your iron intake (see Tip, below).

• • •

MAKES 2 PORTIONS

2 tablespoons chopped mango chutney

1 tablespoon whole-grain Dijon mustard

2 tablespoons Worcestershire sauce

4 skinless, boneless chicken thighs

Salt and pepper

1 tablespoon olive oil

Sticky chicken thighs

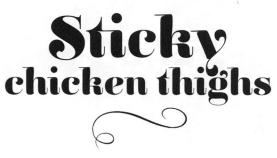

✶ RICH IN IRON ✶

✶ Mix the chutney, mustard, and Worcestershire sauce in a medium bowl. Pound the thighs with a rolling pin so that they are thinner. Add to the marinade and season with salt and pepper. Marinate for 1 hour in the fridge.

✶ Heat the oil in a frying pan. Cook the thighs over medium heat for 10 to 12 minutes, turning halfway through, until golden, sticky, and cooked through.

Tip

Both you and your baby are putting great demands on your iron stores during pregnancy (see page 16). If you're trying to maximize your iron intake, remember that the darker meat of chicken thighs contains more iron than breast meat. It's also higher in zinc.

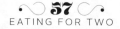

This is real comfort food—a tasty chicken pie in a delicious creamy sauce, topped with cheesy mashed potatoes. It is a great dish to store in the freezer for days when you don't want to cook.

• • •

MAKES 4 PORTIONS
SUITABLE FOR FREEZING

1¼ pounds Yukon Gold potatoes, peeled and cut into chunks
4 tablespoons butter
½ cup milk
½ cup grated Cheddar cheese
3 tablespoons grated Parmesan cheese
1 leek, white and pale green parts only, thinly sliced
1 large or 2 small shallots, finely chopped
3 tablespoons all-purpose flour
1¼ cups chicken broth
½ cup heavy cream
4 cups (loosely packed) shredded cooked chicken
⅔ cup frozen peas
1 tablespoon chopped fresh parsley
1 tablespoon lemon juice
Salt and pepper

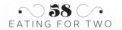

Tasty chicken and potato pie

✳ Put the potatoes in cold salted water, bring to a boil, then reduce the heat and simmer for 10 to 15 minutes, until tender. Drain and mash with 2 tablespoons of the butter, the milk, and the grated Cheddar and Parmesan.

✳ Preheat the oven to 400°F.

✳ Melt the remaining 2 tablespoons butter in a saucepan and cook the leek and shallot gently for 8 to 10 minutes, until soft but not colored. Stir in the flour and cook for 1 minute, then stir in the broth a little at a time to make a smooth sauce (you may find it easier to do this off the heat).

✳ Stir in the cream, then cook, stirring, until the sauce just comes to a boil. Stir in the chicken, peas, and parsley, then remove from the heat and stir in the lemon juice. Season with salt and pepper to taste. Spoon into a 1½-quart (8 × 8-inch) dish and top with the mashed potatoes. It's a good idea to place the dish on a baking sheet to catch any drips. Bake for about 30 minutes or until golden brown (it will need longer if cooking from frozen; check that it's piping hot all the way through).

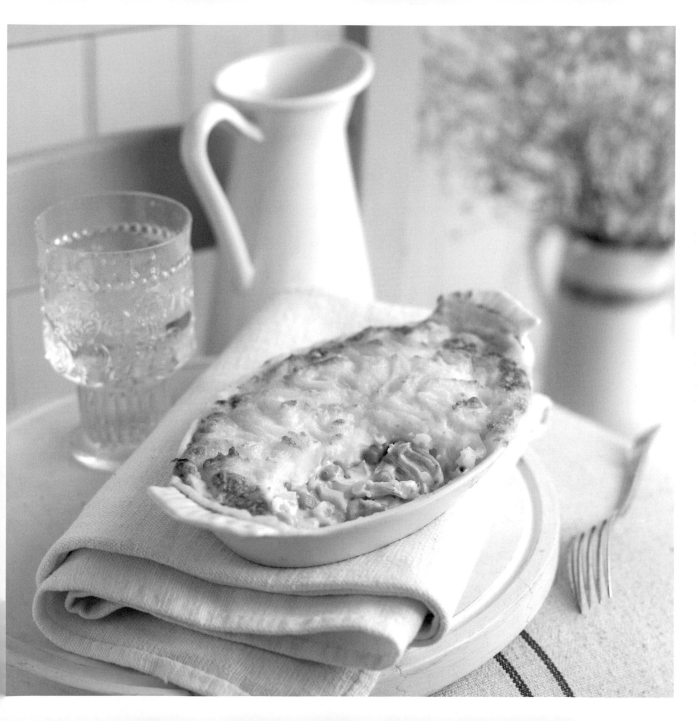

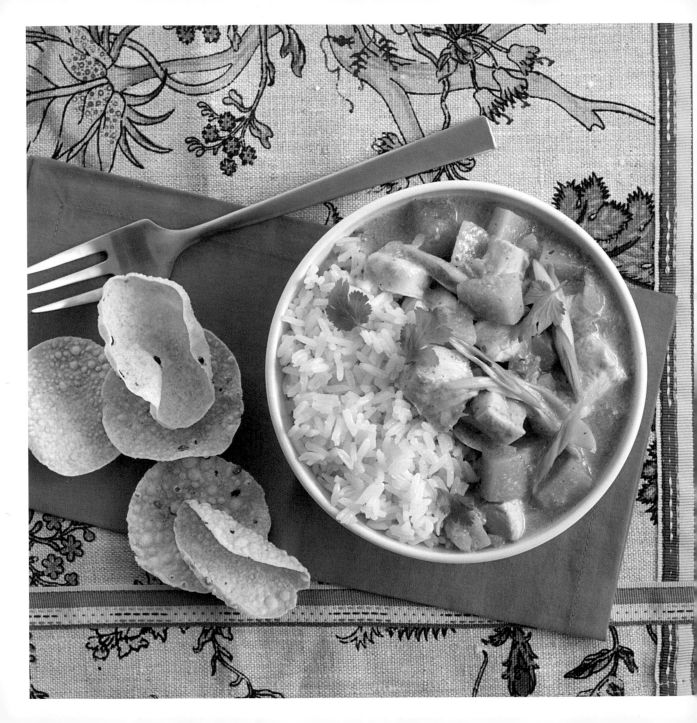

This is one of my favorite chicken recipes. I love the combination of the creamy coconut and red curry paste and the tender pieces of chicken and diced butternut squash.

...

Thai chicken
with butternut squash

MAKES 2 PORTIONS
SUITABLE FOR FREEZING

2 tablespoons canola oil
2 onions, sliced
½-inch piece fresh ginger, peeled and grated
1 clove garlic, crushed
2 tablespoons Thai red curry paste
1½ tablespoons all-purpose flour
One 13.5-ounce can coconut milk
1¼ cups chicken broth or water
2 to 3 teaspoons fish sauce (nam pla)
2 teaspoons brown sugar
Zest and juice of half a lime
½ lemongrass stalk, white part only, pounded
Scant 1 cup diced peeled butternut squash
2 skinless, boneless chicken breasts, cubed
2 scallions, sliced, for garnish
Fresh cilantro, for garnish

✴ Heat 1 tablespoon of the oil in a saucepan. Add the onions, ginger, and garlic and gently sauté for 8 to 10 minutes, until soft. Add the curry paste and flour and cook for 1 minute.

✴ Blend in the coconut milk, broth or water, fish sauce, sugar, and lime zest and juice. Bring to a boil and simmer for 5 minutes.

✴ Add the lemongrass and the butternut squash, cover with a lid, and simmer for another 5 minutes.

✴ Heat the remaining 1 tablespoon oil in a frying pan. Brown the chicken, then add to the sauce and simmer for 5 to 6 minutes, until cooked through. Remove the lemongrass.

✴ Serve with jasmine rice and mini pappadams. Garnish with scallions and fresh cilantro.

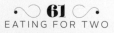

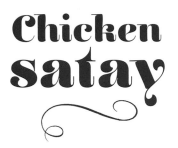

Chicken satay

2 cloves garlic, peeled
1 tablespoon chopped fresh
ginger
3 tablespoons peanut butter
2 tablespoons rice vinegar
3 tablespoons light soy sauce
3 tablespoons brown sugar
1 small chile, seeded
3 tablespoons lime juice
1 small shallot, peeled
Salt and pepper
2 skinless, boneless chicken
breasts
1 tablespoon peanut oil

To serve:
Sweet chili sauce (optional)

✻ Put all the ingredients except the chicken and peanut oil in a mini food processor and blend until smooth.

✻ Cut the chicken into strips and let marinate in the sauce for at least 30 minutes or up to 4 hours in the fridge; the longer, the better. To cook, heat the peanut oil in a hot frying pan, add the chicken, and sauté until it is cooked through and the surface is caramelized. Alternatively, the chicken can be put on skewers and grilled or broiled. Serve with a dipping sauce, such as sweet chili sauce.

Tip
Unless you are allergic to peanuts, it is safe to eat peanuts and indeed any nuts (see page 28) when you are pregnant.

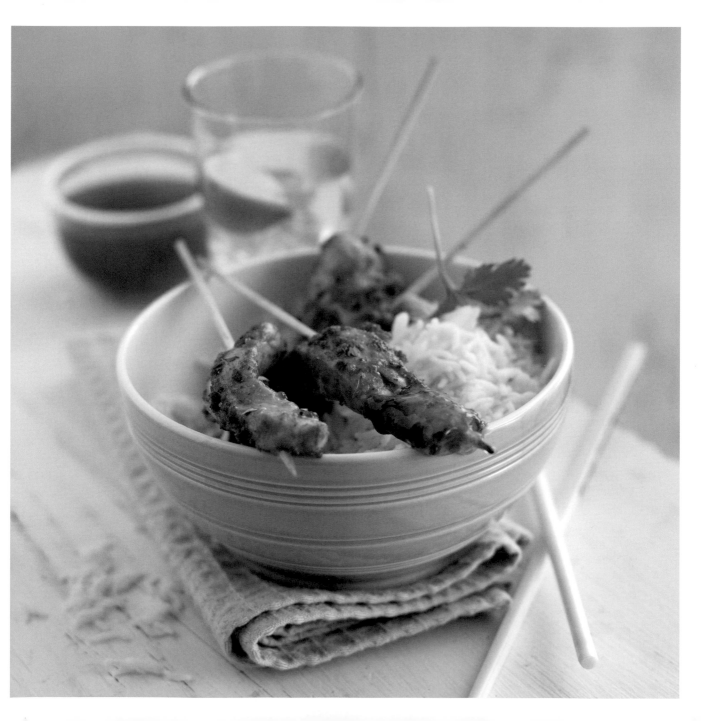

Arugula contains a little of the plant form of omega-3 oils. It also offers iron, calcium, and folic acid.

• • •

Zest and juice of 1 small lemon
Pinch of red pepper flakes
1 clove garlic, crushed
1 tablespoon olive oil
1 teaspoon honey
1 sprig fresh rosemary, finely chopped
2 skinless, boneless chicken breasts
1 large zucchini
1 yellow bell pepper, seeded and sliced into thick wedges
1½ tablespoons olive oil
4 cups (loosely packed) arugula
½ pear, peeled, cored, and thinly sliced
2 tablespoons pine nuts, toasted
1 ounce Parmesan cheese, shaved

Dressing
2 teaspoons Dijon mustard
1 teaspoon rice wine vinegar
2 tablespoons olive oil
1 tablespoon lemon juice
Pinch of sugar

Chicken salad with pears, arugula, and grilled zucchini

✶ Combine the lemon zest and juice, red pepper flakes, garlic, olive oil, honey, and rosemary in a shallow dish and mix together to make the marinade. Put the chicken breasts on a cutting board. Cover with plastic wrap and pound with a rolling pin so they are thinner. Put in the marinade, cover, and refrigerate for 30 minutes to 1 hour.

✶ Slice the zucchini into thin ribbons. Put in a bowl with the bell pepper. Add the olive oil and toss together. Heat a grill pan until hot, then grill the zucchini and bell pepper until soft and golden. Transfer to a mixing bowl and let cool.

✶ Scatter the arugula on a plate. Arrange the zucchini ribbons, yellow bell pepper, and pear on top. Sprinkle with the pine nuts and Parmesan. Make the dressing: Mix the mustard, rice wine vinegar, olive oil, lemon juice, and sugar together in a bowl. Pour onto the salad.

✶ Heat the grill pan. When hot, add the marinated chicken. Cook for 8 to 10 minutes, turning halfway through. Let cool a little, then slice the breasts and arrange on top of the salad.

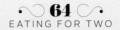

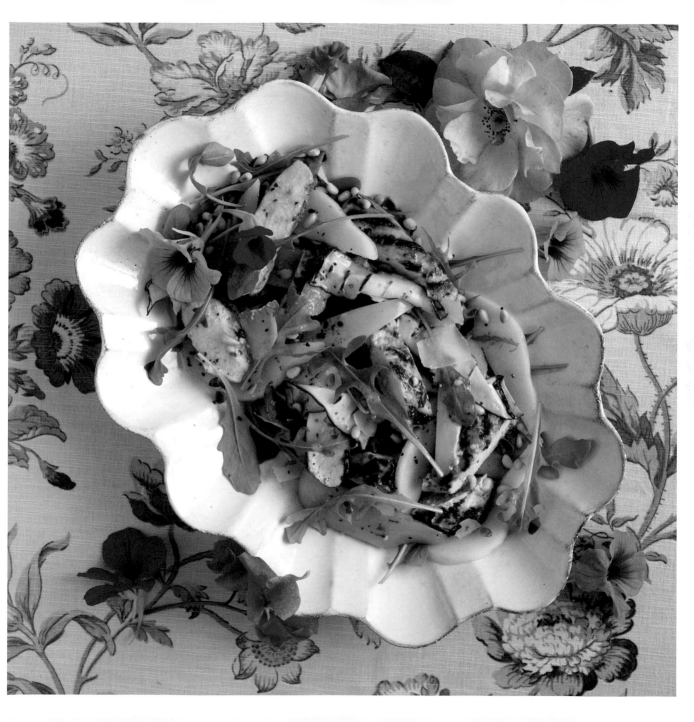

½ cup orange juice
1 clove garlic, crushed
1 teaspoon soy sauce
½ teaspoon grated fresh
 ginger
1 tablespoon honey
2 boneless chicken breasts,
 skin on
1 tablespoon olive oil
⅔ cup chicken broth
1 teaspoon cornstarch
Salt and pepper

Marinated
chicken breasts with
soy-orange sauce

* Combine the orange juice, garlic, soy sauce, ginger, and honey in a bowl. Add the chicken breasts. Cover and marinate in the refrigerator for 4 hours, or overnight if possible.

* Preheat the oven to 400°F.

* Remove the chicken from the marinade. Heat the oil in a frying pan. Cook the chicken, skin side down, until golden, turn over, and cook for another minute. Transfer to a baking sheet and roast for 15 minutes.

* Strain the marinade into the pan. Bring to a boil and reduce by half. Add the broth and reduce again. Mix the cornstarch with a little cold water. Stir into the sauce to thicken. Season with salt and pepper and serve with the chicken. Serve with a green vegetable such as steamed baby bok choy and grilled orange slices.

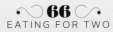

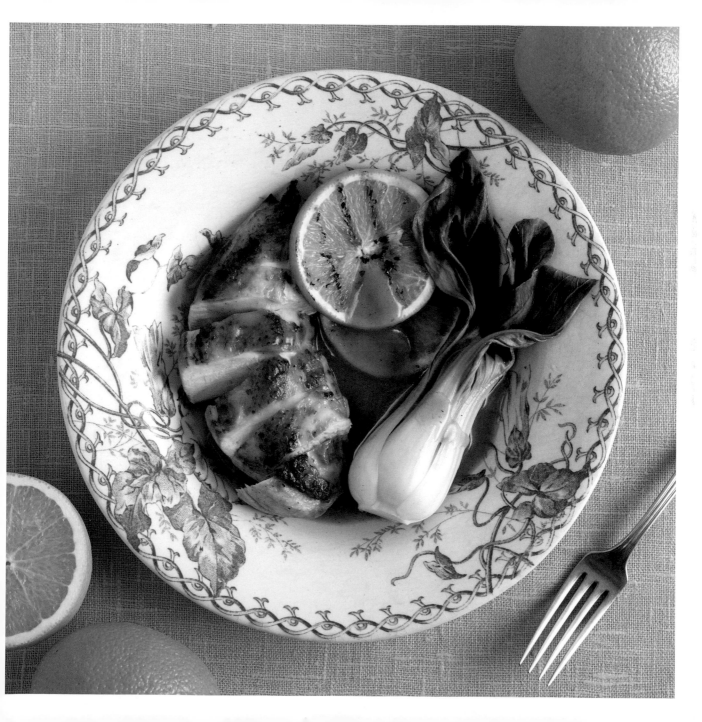

A quesadilla is usually made with one or two flour tortillas. The tortillas are filled with cheese and other ingredients, folded or sandwiched, then griddled until the cheese melts. Traditionally, they are cut into wedges. For more quesadilla recipes, see pages 154 to 156.

• • •

MAKES 1 PORTION

1 tablespoon salsa (good-quality store-bought)
1 large (12-inch) flour tortilla or 2 small (8-inch) tortillas
1 cup (loosely packed) shredded cooked chicken breast
½ cup grated sharp Cheddar
Black pepper (optional)
2 tablespoons guacamole
1 tablespoon sour cream

Chicken
quesadilla

✳ Preheat a large nonstick frying pan over medium-low heat.

✳ Spread the salsa over one half of the large tortilla, or over the whole of one of the tortillas if using the smaller ones. Scatter the chicken and Cheddar on top and season with a little pepper, if desired. Fold over the other half of the tortilla to sandwich in the salsa, chicken, and cheese (or use the second small tortilla to sandwich).

✳ Slide the filled tortilla(s) into the frying pan and cook for 2 to 3 minutes, until golden brown underneath. Carefully flip the quesadilla over and cook for 2 to 3 minutes more, until the cheese has melted and the outside is crisp.

✳ Slide the quesadilla onto a plate and let stand for 2 to 3 minutes (to let the cheese set a little). Cut into 4 to 8 wedges. Serve with the guacamole and sour cream.

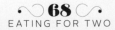

1 tablespoon canola oil

1 onion, chopped

2 cloves garlic, crushed

½-inch piece fresh ginger, peeled and grated

1 red chile, seeded and sliced

1½ to 2 teaspoons mild korma curry paste (such as Patak's)

1 tablespoon brown sugar

One 13.5-ounce can coconut milk

1¼ cups chicken broth or water

2 teaspoons soy sauce

⅔ cup thinly sliced cremini mushrooms

2 ounces green beans, cut into 1-inch pieces

2 cooked chicken breasts, cut into small strips

Grated zest and juice of half a small lime

1 teaspoon fish sauce (nam pla)

2 large scallions, sliced

Salt and pepper

4 ounces thin egg noodles, cooked following package instructions

To garnish (optional):

Small handful of fresh cilantro

Slices of red chile

Chicken
laksa

✶ Heat the oil in a saucepan. Add the onion, garlic, ginger, and chile and sauté for 2 minutes. Add the curry paste, sugar, coconut milk, broth or water, and soy sauce. Bring to a boil. Add the mushrooms, beans, and chicken and simmer for about 5 minutes, until the chicken is cooked through. Add the zest and juice of the lime, fish sauce, scallions, and salt and pepper to taste.

✶ Divide the noodles among three bowls and add the soup. Garnish with cilantro and chile slices, if using.

Tip
Some pregnant women find that foods containing ginger help to relieve morning sickness. Ginger also adds a delicious, fresh flavor to food.

3: The Second Trimester

The Second Trimester: Full of life
This trimester often marks the most enjoyable time of pregnancy. Morning sickness should be a memory, or at least much improved, and energy levels often increase. Some women even experience a surge in libido! It's a time when your baby's growth rate increases—he may triple his length during these three months—and you'll experience the excitement of feeling him move. Your diet supports a long list of developmental milestones, from your baby's bones beginning to form to his beginning to hear and possibly respond to your voice. So please continue to eat well, for both of you.

Nutrition priorities during the second trimester
For many women, this trimester sees a surge in appetite. The focus can change from eating sufficient calories and nutrients to trying to control a sometimes ravenous appetite, possibly for less healthy foods. Eating more than you require, and gaining excess weight, can result in a bigger baby, as well as increasing the risk of developing diabetes during pregnancy. Read on for more tips on managing appetite during the second trimester.

With your baby developing bones and body organs such as his eyes and ears, and both of you gaining weight, your need for nutrients has never been greater. Continue to follow the balanced diet outlined in chapter 1. This will ensure you're getting the calcium, protein, iron, and other nutrients crucial to this trimester.

This is likely to be the time for a wardrobe makeover—you'll notice a (sometimes dramatic) midline expansion that will put your favorite jeans out of action for the time being. This trimester may also signal the beginning of such unglamorous issues as constipation. Read on for more on managing this and the change in body image that can go hand in hand with your blossoming figure.

You and your baby during the second trimester

You
Your heart is beating an amazing extra 14,000 beats each day.

• • •

Energy levels are often up in the second trimester, but don't be tempted to skip meals. Regular meals and snacks are still essential.

• • •

If you began your pregnancy within your healthy weight range, a healthy weight gain is about 3 to 4 pounds per month in the second and third trimesters.

Your baby
Your baby is still developing, and now his rate of growth increases. By 20 weeks he can kick his legs, wave his arms, and grasp with his fists.

• • •

Your baby needs calcium to develop strong bones and teeth. A good supply of protein is also crucial at this time of rapid growth.

• • •

By week 24 your baby measures about 9 inches and weighs less than 2.2 pounds.

Nutritional issues
Food, glorious food
If you battled morning sickness in the first trimester, the increased appetite of the second trimester can

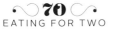

come as a relief. However, it can be a mixed blessing—while you might find it easier to eat all the foods your body and your baby need, you might also find yourself wanting to eat extra calories or having trouble resisting less healthy options. If this is a problem, start by planning your daily intake. Make sure you are fitting in all the foods required from the food groups, so you are getting your required nutrients. You could indulge yourself with a treat every once in a while—resisting too much can just make it worse. However, if you find yourself having too many extras, here are some helpful hints:

* Eat regularly and don't skip meals. Plan meals and snacks to avoid getting overly hungry and eating more than you might otherwise.
* Be organized. If you have a healthy snack with you, you'll be much less likely to grab a chocolate bar at the supermarket checkout. See page 31 for a list of healthy, portable snacks.
* Fill up with fiber. Choose foods that are higher in fiber to keep you fuller and reduce hunger pangs—see more on this on page 13.
* Go for a low GI. The glycemic index (otherwise known as GI) is a measure of how slowly the carbohydrates, or fuel, in food are made available to the body during digestion. Foods with a low GI will be digested slowly, and some studies show that they fill people up more. Higher GI foods are used up more quickly and theoretically keep you filled and fueled for a shorter time. GI is often related to the amount of fiber in a food, but it's more complex than that.

For example, chocolate has a low GI, but is not high in fiber. Nor is it a healthy choice, which shows

that you do need to think about more th[...] Particularly low GI foods that are also healthy options include oat-based foods such as oatmeal, granola, and muesli, as well as bean- or legume-based foods such as lentil soup or baked beans. Choosing lower GI foods (see below) a few times each day may help to control those hunger pangs.

* Drink up. Make sure you are drinking enough fluids. Some people go looking for a snack when it's actually a drink their bodies are after.

Top 10: Filling (and nutritious) snacks
* Toasted fruit bread with reduced-fat cream cheese and jam
* Mix of nuts and dried fruit
* Fresh apple with a wedge of reduced-fat cheese
* Bowl of high-fiber breakfast cereal with low-fat milk
* Multigrain crispbread with hummus
* Smoothie made with low-fat milk, banana, and strawberries
* Low-fat nutrition bar
* Bowl of chopped fresh fruit topped with reduced-fat plain yogurt, a sprinkle of crunchy granola, and a drizzle of honey
* Cup of lentil soup
* Canned salmon mixed with reduced-fat cream cheese and a squeeze of lemon juice, atop a toasted English muffin (preferably whole-grain)

Top 10: Low-GI foods
* Oatmeal, muesli, and multigrain crispbread
* Whole-grain bread and tortillas
* Apples, pears, and grapes
* Peaches, plums, and oranges
* Pasta made from durum wheat, and noodles

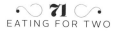

..., peas, and lentils, including

..., carrots, and corn

...ati rice

Can a special diet help you sleep?

Having trouble sleeping is a common complaint in pregnancy, partly due to aches and pains and partly due to hormonal highs and lows. Some people swear by warm milk to help them drift off, others by eating turkey, but does any food really help?

While the role of turkey in helping people sleep has little to back it up scientifically, one study found that a meal with a high glycemic index (GI) about four hours before bedtime could reduce the time taken to fall asleep. High-GI foods include white bread and baguettes, white rice (not basmati), parsnips, watermelon, rice cakes, and mashed and baked potatoes. You can read more about GI on page 71.

One more tip: You'll already be limiting the amount of caffeine you consume from tea, coffee, and cola, but try to avoid having any caffeinated drinks in the late afternoon and the evening if you're having trouble drifting off.

Constipation

Constipation is a frequent problem during pregnancy: After all, by the later stages, there is a whole baby resting on your large intestine! Earlier on, however, problems can occur because the pregnancy hormones relax the muscles of the intestine, meaning that they don't move the matter inside along so efficiently. Constipation increases the chance of developing another dreaded pregnancy issue—hemorrhoids—so it shouldn't be ignored.

Many people think constipation can be sorted out simply by adding fiber to the diet, but there is more to it. Fiber, found in grain foods, fruit and vegetables, legumes, and nuts and seeds, needs additional fluid to help it work. Keeping active also helps your muscles to move things along. However, sometimes this problem cannot be solved with food, drink, and activity alone. If you've tried all the tips below and are still having problems, talk to your ob-gyn, because medication could be required.

Top 10 ways to beat constipation

* Drink a glass of fluid (water is a great choice, but any nonalcoholic drink will do) with every meal and snack, plus another couple for good measure. Water combines with fiber to create softer, bulkier stools that are easier to pass. While drinks that contain caffeine do count toward your fluid intake, remember that they should be limited during pregnancy.
* Stay active: A little exercise, even a gentle stroll, helps keep everything moving along.
* Whole-grain foods are a great source of fiber. Choose these over the more refined, "white" varieties. They include multigrain bread, whole-grain breakfast cereal, brown rice, whole wheat pasta, and whole-grain couscous.
* Fruit is a tasty place to find fiber. Serve fruit unpeeled (though washed thoroughly) where possible, to gain extra fiber. A handful of chopped dried fruit is a great addition to breakfast cereal, yogurt, or dessert.

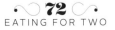

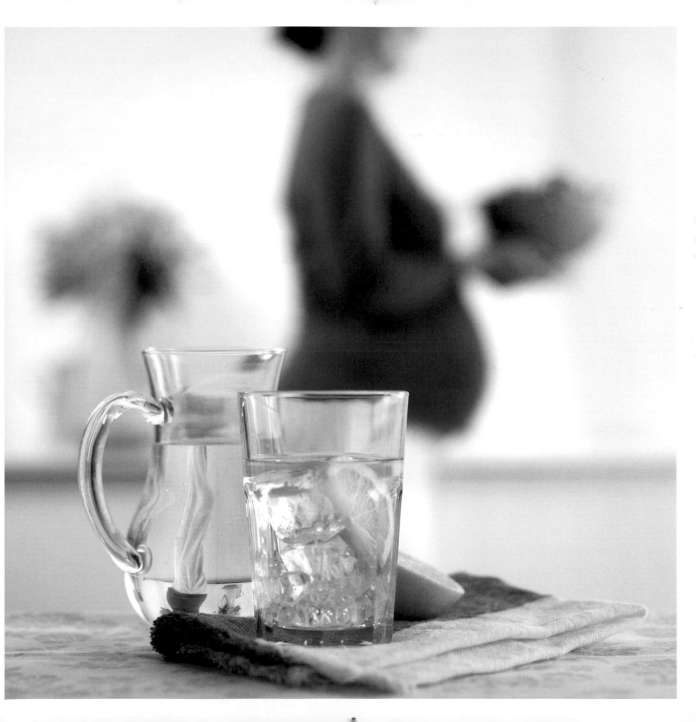

* Vegetables: Fill sandwiches with (thoroughly washed) greens, and remember to include vegetables or a salad at your evening meal. Frozen vegetables are a convenient choice and can be just as nutritious as fresh.
* Dried beans, chickpeas, and lentils: Eating baked beans, bean salad, and lentil soup will increase your intake of these fiber-rich foods. You could also add canned beans to soups and stews.
* Nuts and seeds: Sprinkle some nuts or seeds on salads, breakfast cereal, oatmeal, or desserts. You could snack on a dried fruit and nut mix.
* Prunes and prune juice: These contain a substance that gently helps the bowels to move. Try adding some prunes or a glass or two of prune juice to your diet for a few days to see if it helps.
* Consider your iron supplement: Many women use iron supplements during pregnancy, and some can contribute to constipation. Perhaps talk to your pharmacist about trying a different type.
* Fiber supplements: If you're still having problems with constipation after looking at fluid intake, exercise, and fiber, speak to your ob-gyn or pharmacist.

Body image

For the many women who keep a close check on their weight, the rapid expansion of pregnancy can be difficult to deal with. From forgetting how big you physically are (until you try to edge through a just-too-small gap between café tables) to catching sight of a new, larger you in a mirror, there are times when you are unexpectedly confronted with the weight gain some women fear. If you are finding this

difficult, spend some time reading over the nutrition information in chapter 1. Remember how much the nutrients in the foods you eat are benefiting your baby, and that the weight you are gaining is essential to support him. Reassure yourself with the weight gain guidelines that the pounds you're gaining are normal and necessary. If you are still worried, talk to your health care provider. Under no circumstances should you try to eat fewer calories to keep weight gain below recommended levels.

If you are gaining weight faster than the recommended 3 to 4 pounds a month, you could also read over the advice on higher-fat and higher-sugar foods in chapter 1 (see page 15) and the information on controlling appetite on pages 70 to 71.

Pregnancy Myth Buster: Do cravings mean our body is missing nutrients?

Mention a craving during pregnancy and you're likely to be told that it's your body's way of getting you to eat a nutrient you're missing. Can this really be true? Scientists are generally skeptical; however, they have done some research into pica. This is the desire to eat substances, such as clay or match heads, that aren't food. Scientists have found that many people with pica have low iron levels, but whether this is the cause of the craving is debatable. Researchers are divided into those who believe the pica is caused by iron deficiency and those who think the deficiency is caused by the pica. This could happen because some of the unusual substances eaten bind to the iron in the digestive system and prevent its being absorbed. One thing is certain: If you have an overwhelming desire of this type, talk to your health care provider.

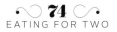

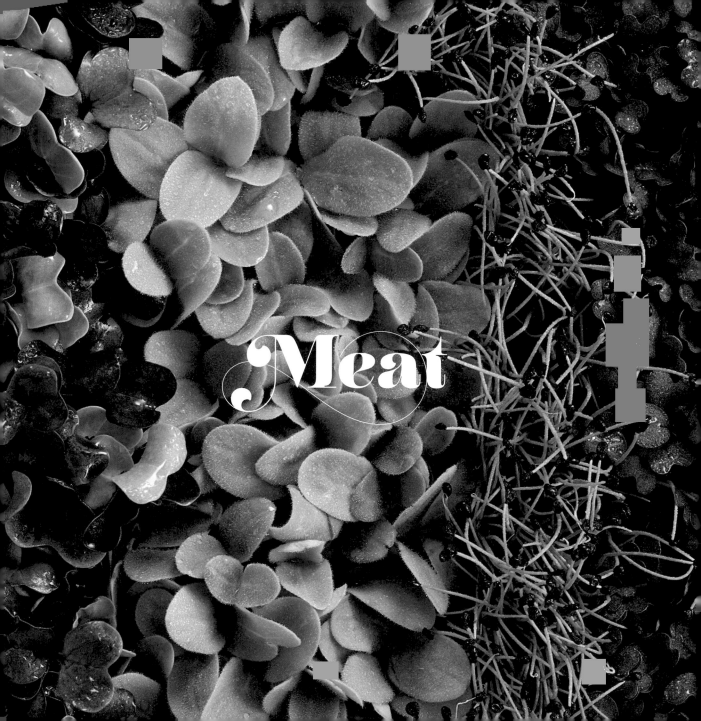

3 tablespoons canola oil
1 pound beef stew meat, diced
1 large onion, chopped
2 cloves garlic, crushed
1 teaspoon ground cumin
1 teaspoon ground coriander
1 teaspoon ground ginger
½ teaspoon ground cinnamon
5 dried apricots, chopped
1 teaspoon honey
One 14-ounce can diced tomatoes
1 cup beef broth
1 teaspoon tomato paste
Half a 15-ounce can chickpeas, drained and rinsed
Juice of half a lemon

Beef tagine

✱ RICH IN IRON ✱

✱ Preheat the oven to 350°F.

✱ Heat 2 tablespoons of the oil in a frying pan. Brown the beef in batches. Heat the remaining 1 tablespoon oil in a saucepan or casserole dish, add the onion and garlic, and sauté for 4 minutes. Add the beef and mix together. Sprinkle with the spices, apricots, and honey and sauté for 1 minute. Blend in the tomatoes, broth, and tomato paste. Bring to a boil, cover, and transfer to the oven for 1½ to 2 hours, or until the beef is tender. Ten minutes before the end of the cooking time, add the chickpeas and lemon juice.

✱ Serve with couscous.

Tip:

Including iron-rich foods in your diet will reduce your chance of becoming anemic and needing iron supplements—a common problem when pregnant. Red meat provides the best and most easily absorbed source of iron during pregnancy.

I love really thin steak, and the beauty of it is that it takes only minutes to cook. Try it with this lovely caramelized onion gravy.

• • •

MAKES 2 PORTIONS

Two 6-ounce sandwich
    (minute) steaks
Pat of butter, softened
Salt and pepper
1 tablespoon canola oil
1 onion, thinly sliced
½ teaspoon brown sugar
2 teaspoons all-purpose
    flour
1 cup beef broth
1 to 1½ teaspoons balsamic
    vinegar
1½ teaspoons
    Worcestershire sauce
1 teaspoon chopped fresh
    thyme leaves

Minute steaks with onion and thyme gravy

✳ Put the sandwich steaks on a cutting board. Cover with plastic wrap and pound, using a rolling pin, to ½-inch thickness. Spread the butter over the steaks and season with salt and pepper.

✳ Heat a frying pan until hot. Fry the steaks for 1 minute on each side, or until cooked through, then transfer to a warm plate and cover with foil.

✳ Add the oil to the pan and sauté the onion over medium heat until softened. Add the sugar and brown the onion. Sprinkle with the flour, then blend in the broth. Add the balsamic vinegar, Worcestershire sauce, and thyme, and season with salt and pepper. Stir until thickened and simmer for 2 minutes, or until reduced slightly. Add any juices from the steaks to the gravy.

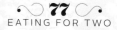

2 tablespoons mirin
2 tablespoons soy sauce
2 tablespoons hoisin sauce
1 tablespoon water
1 tablespoon cornstarch
8 ounces top loin, shell steak, or New York strip steak, thinly sliced
2 tablespoons Asian sesame oil
2 teaspoons honey
Salt and pepper
Handful of small broccoli florets
½ red bell pepper, seeded and cut into strips
6 ears baby corn, halved lengthwise
1 cup sugar snap peas, strings removed (optional)
1 baby bok choy, separated into leaves

Tender beef stir-fry

✻ LOW FAT ✻

✳ Mix the mirin, soy sauce, hoisin sauce, water, and cornstarch together in a small bowl until smooth.

✳ Heat a wok until hot. Coat the steak slices with 1 tablespoon of the sesame oil and the honey and season with salt and pepper. Quickly stir-fry over high heat until browned and just cooked. Transfer to a plate.

✳ Heat the remaining 1 tablespoon sesame oil in the wok. Add the broccoli and bell pepper and stir-fry for 3 minutes. Add the corn and sugar snap peas, if using, and stir-fry for another 2 minutes. Pour in the sauce and season with salt and pepper to taste. Add the bok choy and then the steak slices. Toss together until the sauce has coated the vegetables and beef.

✳ Serve at once with rice or noodles.

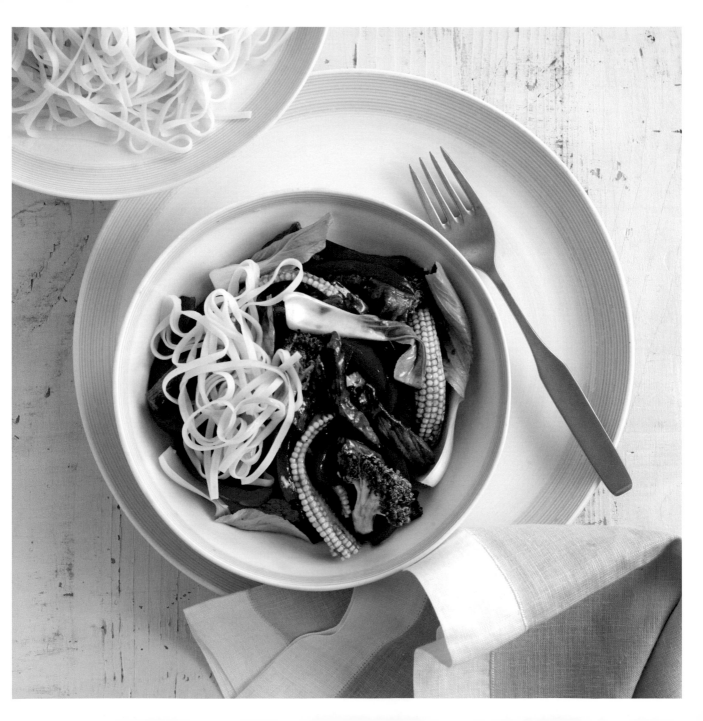

1 tablespoon canola oil

1¼ pounds beef stew meat, diced

1 large onion, sliced

1 red bell pepper, seeded and thickly sliced

2 cloves garlic, crushed

1 tablespoon paprika

1½ tablespoons tomato paste

1⅔ cups beef broth

1½ teaspoons balsamic vinegar

½ teaspoon brown sugar

½ teaspoon soy sauce

⅓ cup crème fraîche or sour cream

Hungarian
goulash

✳ Preheat the oven to 350°F.

✳ Heat the oil in an oven-safe frying pan. Brown the beef on all sides until golden, then transfer to a plate. Add the onion to the pan with the bell pepper and sauté for 3 to 4 minutes. Add the garlic, paprika, and tomato paste and cook for 2 minutes more. Return the beef to the pan and coat in the onion mixture. Add the broth and bring to a boil. Cover with a lid and place in the oven for 1 hour. Remove from the oven and add the remaining ingredients. Bring back to a boil, cover, and return to the oven for 30 to 40 minutes, until the beef is tender.

✳ Serve with rice or mashed potatoes.

Tip:
Tea and coffee contain substances that make it harder for your body to absorb iron, so try not to have a mug of your favorite brew with your meal or immediately after it.

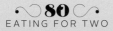

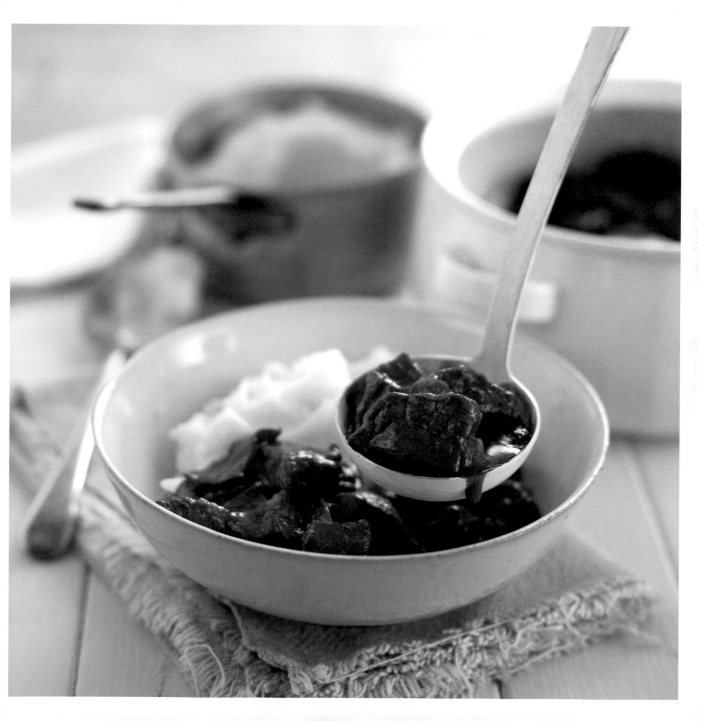

This classic Russian dish is one of my favorites. It's usually made with button mushrooms, but you could use shiitake mushrooms instead. Serve with rice or thick noodles.

• • •

Beef stroganoff

MAKES 2 OR 3 PORTIONS

2 tablespoons butter

1 tablespoon olive oil

12 ounces beef tenderloin, sliced into 6 thick strips

Salt and pepper

2 small onions, finely chopped

2 cups thinly sliced button mushrooms

5 tablespoons white wine

5 tablespoons good-quality beef broth

1 tablespoon Dijon mustard

1 tablespoon Worcestershire sauce

Scant 1 cup crème fraîche or heavy cream

1 teaspoon lemon juice

2 tablespoons chopped fresh parsley

✴ Heat a frying pan until hot. Add 1 tablespoon of the butter and the oil. Season the beef with salt and pepper, then quickly brown, until just cooked, over high heat. Transfer to a plate.

✴ Add the remaining 1 tablespoon butter to the pan. Sauté the onions for 5 minutes, or until just softened, then add the mushrooms and sauté for 2 minutes more. Pour in the wine and broth and reduce by half. Add the Dijon mustard and Worcestershire sauce and simmer for 30 seconds. Pour in the crème fraîche and lemon juice and bring to a boil. Add the beef and warm through. Stir in the parsley and serve at once with rice or noodles.

MAKES 6 BURGERS
SUITABLE FOR FREEZING

1 cup fresh bread crumbs
8 ounces lean ground beef
1 large red onion, finely
  chopped
2 teaspoons Dijon mustard
1 teaspoon tomato paste
1 tablespoon Worcestershire
  sauce
1 teaspoon soy sauce
½ cup grated Parmesan
  cheese
1 tablespoon chopped fresh
  thyme
Salt and pepper

To fry:
All-purpose flour, to coat
2 tablespoons canola oil

To broil:
Pat of butter

Annabel's hamburgers

✳ Put all of the burger ingredients except the salt and pepper in a food processor and whiz until just combined. Transfer to a bowl, season with salt and pepper, and shape into 6 patties.

✳ To fry: Lightly coat the patties with flour. Heat the oil in a large frying pan and fry the patties for 3 to 4 minutes on each side, until golden and cooked through.

✳ To broil: Preheat the broiler and line the broiler pan with foil. Place the patties on the broiler pan, dot with a little butter, and broil for about 5 minutes on each side, or until cooked through.

Tip

Dishes that contain ground meat (e.g., burgers and sausages) must be cooked thoroughly so that there's no trace of pink meat or juice.

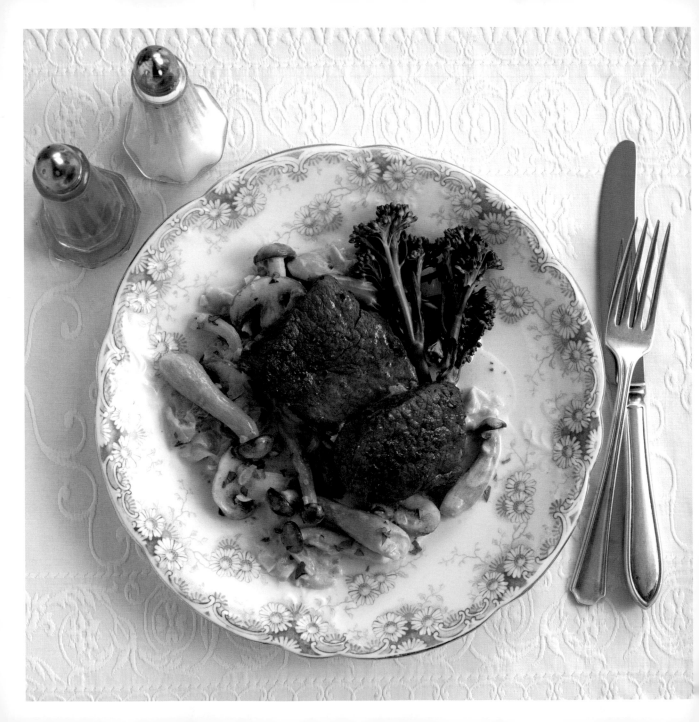

Your unborn baby places huge demands on your iron reserves. If you feel exhausted or dizzy during your pregnancy, you could be suffering from low iron levels. Red meat provides the best source of iron.

• • •

MAKES 2 PORTIONS

2 tablespoons olive oil
Two 1-inch-thick filet mignon steaks (about 5 ounces each)
Salt and pepper
Pat of butter
2 shallots, finely chopped
½ cup white wine
⅓ cup crème fraîche or heavy cream
2 cups mixed wild mushrooms, such as shiitake, oyster, and cremini, halved or sliced if large
3 sprigs fresh tarragon, finely chopped
Pinch of sugar (optional)

Filet mignon
with wild mushroom and tarragon sauce

✷ Heat a large frying pan until hot. Drizzle 1 tablespoon of the oil over the steaks and season well with salt and pepper. Fry the steaks for 2½ to 3 minutes on each side, until cooked through. Transfer to a plate to rest while you make the sauce.

✷ Add the remaining 1 tablespoon oil and the butter to the pan. Add the shallots and sauté for 2 minutes, or until starting to soften. Pour in the wine and reduce by half over high heat. Stir in the crème fraîche. Bring to a boil, then add the mushrooms. Simmer for a few minutes, or until the mushrooms are just cooked, season well with salt and pepper, then add the tarragon and sugar if the sauce tastes a little sharp. Add any juices from the steaks to the pan. Serve the mushroom sauce with the steaks.

Beef fajitas

2 top loin, shell, or New York strip
  steaks (about 10 ounces each)
2 tablespoons canola oil
1 teaspoon ground cumin
½ teaspoon paprika
¼ teaspoon ground coriander
1 clove garlic, crushed
Leaves from 2 sprigs fresh
  thyme, or a pinch of dried
  thyme
1 large red onion, thinly sliced
½ red bell pepper, seeded and
  thinly sliced
½ yellow bell pepper, seeded and
  thinly sliced
½ orange bell pepper, seeded and
  thinly sliced
6 to 8 drops Tabasco sauce
4 to 6 drops Worcestershire sauce
1½ teaspoons brown sugar
Salt and pepper
Juice of half a lime

Avocado relish
1 avocado, peeled and diced
1 tablespoon chopped fresh cilantro
Juice of half a lime
Salt and pepper

To serve:
8 flour tortillas
Store-bought salsa
⅔ cup sour cream

✳ Trim the fat from the steaks, cover them with plastic wrap, and pound with a rolling pin until ¼ inch thick. Cut into thin strips about 1¼ inches long.

✳ In a bowl, mix 1 tablespoon of the oil, the cumin, paprika, coriander, garlic, and thyme. Add the beef, toss to coat, and marinate for 30 minutes in the fridge. Make the avocado relish while the beef marinates.

✳ Heat the remaining 1 tablespoon oil in a wok or large frying pan. Add the onion and bell peppers and stir-fry for 6 to 8 minutes, until soft and slightly charred. Transfer to a plate. Reheat the pan and stir-fry the marinated beef for 2 to 3 minutes, until browned and cooked through. Return the peppers and onion to the pan and stir in the Tabasco, Worcestershire sauce, and sugar. Remove from the heat and season with salt and pepper, then add the lime juice.

✳ To make the relish, mix the avocado and cilantro together. Stir in the lime juice and season with salt and pepper.

✳ To serve, warm the tortillas in the microwave or a dry frying pan. Spoon a little of the beef mixture into the center of each tortilla, top with avocado relish, salsa, and sour cream, and roll up.

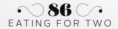

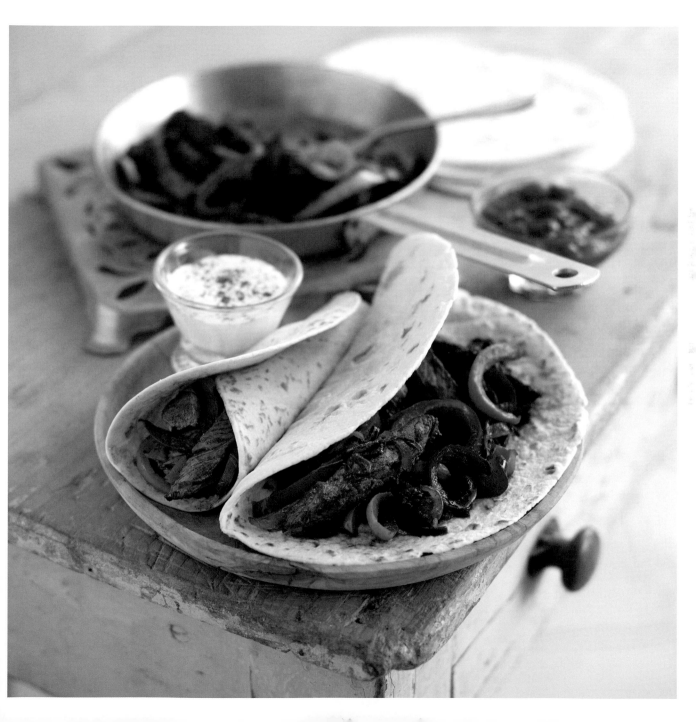

Mixing beef and pork together to make these meatballs keeps them lovely and light. You can use ground chicken instead of the pork if you prefer.

• • •

MAKES 3 OR 4 PORTIONS
SUITABLE FOR FREEZING

4 ounces ground beef
4 ounces ground pork
3 tablespoons grated
    Parmesan cheese
3 tablespoons fresh white
    bread crumbs
1 egg yolk
¾ teaspoon ground
    coriander
Salt and pepper
1 tablespoon olive oil
1 onion, chopped
½ teaspoon grated fresh
    ginger
1 small clove garlic, crushed
½ teaspoon garam masala
⅔ cup chicken broth
One 14-ounce can diced
    tomatoes
1½ teaspoons honey
1 teaspoon tomato paste

Meatballs
in a tagine sauce

✴ Mix together the ground beef, ground pork, Parmesan cheese, bread crumbs, egg yolk, and ¼ teaspoon of the coriander and season with salt and pepper. Shape into 12 balls.

✴ Heat the oil in a saucepan. Add the onion and sauté for 5 minutes. Add the ginger, garlic, the remaining ½ teaspoon coriander, and the garam masala. Stir in the broth, tomatoes, honey, and tomato paste; bring to a boil and simmer for 15 minutes. Transfer to a blender, blend until smooth, then return to the saucepan. Drop in the meatballs and simmer, covered, for 10 minutes, or until the meatballs are cooked through.

✴ Serve with rice.

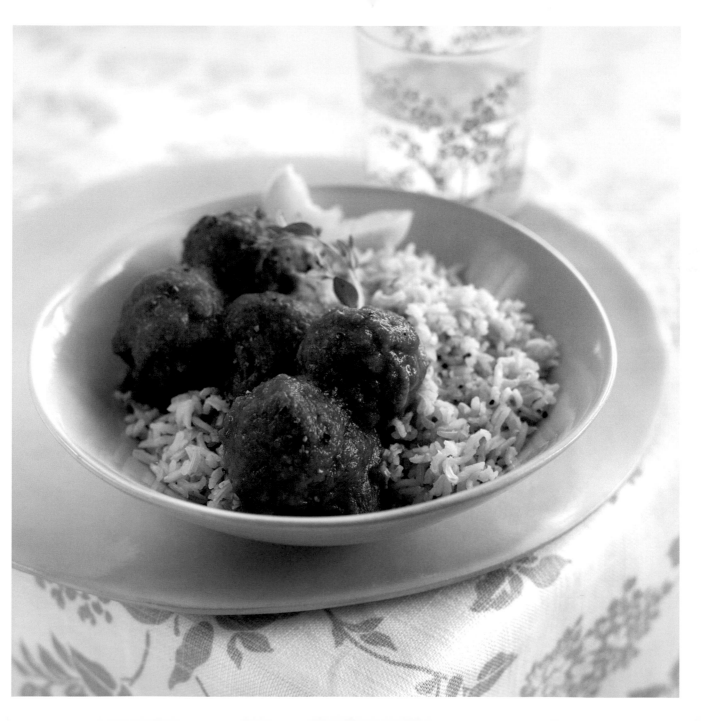

Cannellini beans contain valuable iron, and eating them with lamb, a red meat, will enhance the absorption of the iron.

• • •

MAKES 2 PORTIONS

One 12-ounce frenched rack of lamb

2 tablespoons olive oil

Salt and pepper

4 teaspoons chopped fresh thyme

1 onion, finely chopped

1 clove garlic, crushed

One 15-ounce can cannellini beans, drained and rinsed

One 14-ounce can diced tomatoes

2 teaspoons tomato paste

1 teaspoon Worcestershire sauce

1 teaspoon sugar

3 tablespoons chopped fresh basil

Roast rack of lamb with tomato-and-basil beans

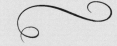

✳ RICH IN IRON ✳

✳ Preheat the oven to 425°F.

✳ Trim all the fat from the rack of lamb. Brush the lamb with 1 tablespoon of the oil, season with salt and pepper, then rub with 3 teaspoons of the thyme. Heat a frying pan until hot. Brown the lamb on both sides for 1½ minutes, then place on a baking sheet. Roast for 10 to 12 minutes. Cover with foil and roast for 5 minutes more, until cooked through.

✳ Heat the remaining 1 tablespoon oil in a saucepan. Add the onion and sauté for 5 minutes, or until softened. Add the garlic and cook for 2 minutes. Add the beans, tomatoes, tomato paste, Worcestershire sauce, and sugar. Bring to a boil and simmer for 10 minutes. Add the remaining 1 teaspoon thyme and the basil and season with salt and pepper to taste.

✳ Carve the lamb and serve with the tomato-and-basil beans.

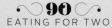

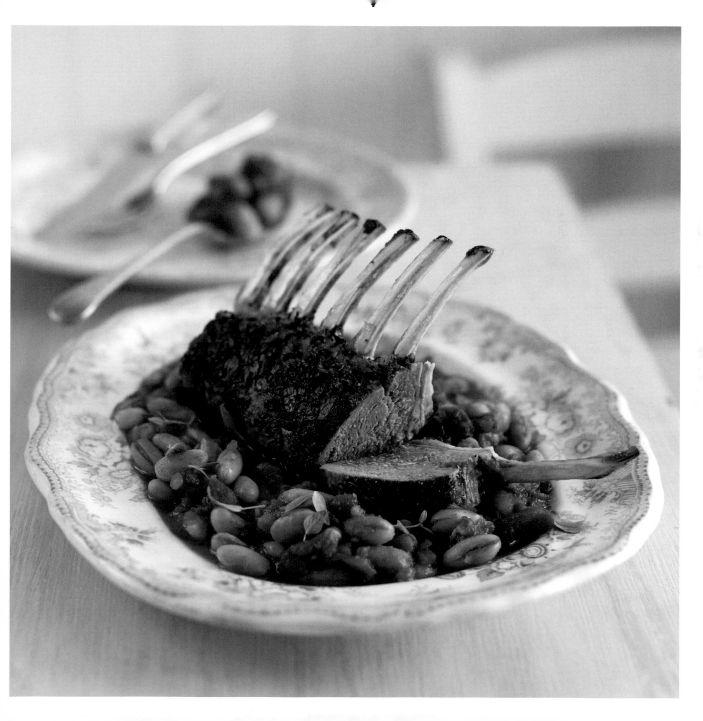

½ teaspoon ground
   coriander
1 cup fresh bread crumbs
1 onion, finely chopped
8 ounces ground lean lamb
¼ cup chopped fresh mint
1 egg yolk
1 teaspoon Dijon mustard
½ teaspoon Worcestershire
   sauce
½ teaspoon lemon juice
Salt and pepper
1 yellow bell pepper, seeded
   and chopped into
   12 pieces
2 tablespoons canola oil

Lamb
kofta kebabs

∗ Put all the ingredients except the salt and pepper, yellow bell pepper, and oil in a food processor. Whiz until just combined. Transfer to a bowl and season with salt and pepper.

∗ Shape into 18 balls. Thread one ball onto a skewer, then a piece of yellow pepper, then another ball, another piece of yellow pepper, and another ball, so you have 3 koftas and 2 pieces of yellow pepper on each of 6 skewers. Refrigerate for 1 hour.

∗ Heat the oil in a frying pan. Fry the kebabs for 10 minutes, or until golden brown and cooked through.

∗ Serve with a Greek yogurt dressing.

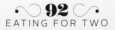

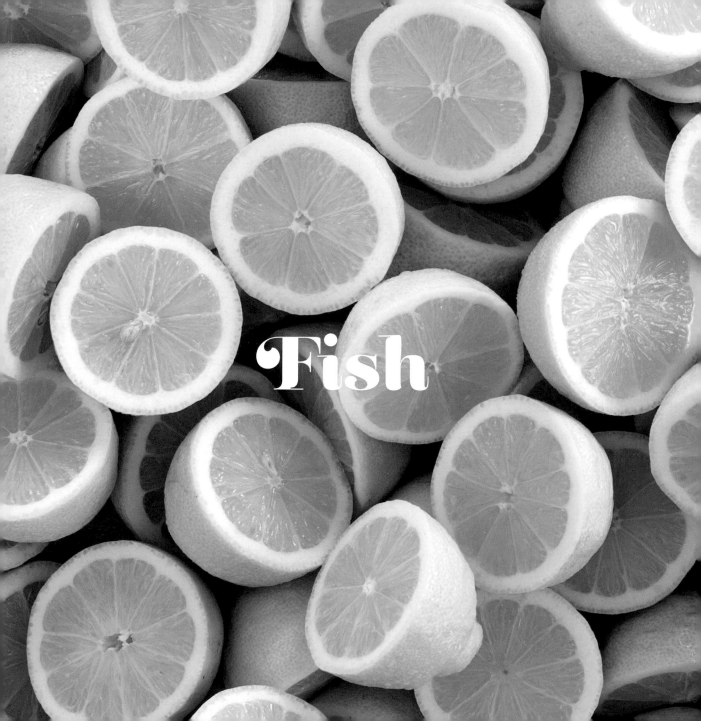

Fish

1½ pounds Yukon Gold
   potatoes, peeled and cut
   into chunks
3 tablespoons milk
Pat of butter

FILLING
3 tablespoons butter
2 shallots, thinly sliced
2 tablespoons rice vinegar
⅓ cup all-purpose flour
1¼ cups fish broth
½ cup heavy cream
1 tablespoon chopped fresh
   chives
1 tablespoon chopped fresh
   dill
¼ cup frozen peas
8 ounces salmon fillet, skin
   removed, sliced into
   pieces
8 ounces cod, skin removed,
   sliced into pieces
¼ cup grated Cheddar
   cheese

Annabel's favorite fish pie

* Preheat the oven to 400°F.

* Cook the potatoes in boiling salted water until tender. Drain and mash with the milk and the pat of butter. Set aside.

* Melt the butter in a saucepan. Add the shallots and sauté for 5 minutes, or until soft. Add the vinegar and stir for 2 minutes. Sprinkle with the flour and stir to make a roux, then blend in the fish broth, stirring until thickened. Add the heavy cream.

* Remove from the heat and add the herbs, peas, and fish. Pour into a shallow ovenproof dish.

* Spread the mashed potatoes over the filling. Sprinkle with the Cheddar.

* Bake for 20 to 25 minutes, until bubbling and lightly golden on top.

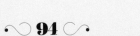

12 ounces potatoes,
    peeled and thinly sliced
1 small onion, sliced
1 teaspoon fresh thyme
    leaves
Salt and pepper
1¼ cups chicken broth
2 branzino fillets, skin on
A little melted butter

Branzino fillets
with sliced potatoes
and thyme

✴ Preheat the oven to 400°F.

✴ Arrange a layer of potatoes on the bottom of a small flameproof dish. Put a few slices of onion on top, sprinkle with the thyme, and season with salt and pepper. Pour over a little broth, then continue to layer until you have used all of the potatoes, onion, and broth.

✴ Cover the dish with foil. Place in the oven for 35 minutes, or until the potatoes are cooked and the broth is bubbling around the edges. Preheat the broiler until hot. Remove the foil and place the dish under the broiler for 5 minutes, or until the potatoes are browned on top.

✴ Season the branzino with salt and pepper and brush with a little melted butter on the skin side of the fillets. Place the fillets (skin side up) on top of the potatoes. Put back under the hot broiler for another 5 minutes, or until the skin is crisp and the fish is cooked through.

¼ cup olive oil
1 small onion, finely
    chopped
1 clove garlic, crushed
1 tablespoon red wine
    vinegar
2 tomatoes, seeded
    and chopped
Pinch of sugar
1 tablespoon finely chopped
    fresh parsley
Salt and pepper
2 red snapper fillets, skin
    on (use branzino if you
    can't get red snapper)
A little all-purpose flour
Lemon wedges or slices,
    to serve (optional)

Red snapper with tomato relish

✳ To make the relish, heat 2 tablespoons of the oil in a small pan. Add the onion and garlic and sauté for 5 to 6 minutes, until soft. Add the vinegar, tomatoes, sugar, and parsley. Warm through for a few minutes, then remove from the heat and season to taste with salt and pepper.

✳ Season the red snapper fillets with salt and pepper and lightly coat with the flour. Heat the remaining 2 tablespoons oil in a frying pan and cook the fish for 2 to 3 minutes on each side, until lightly golden and cooked through.

✳ Serve with the relish and lemon wedges or slices, if using.

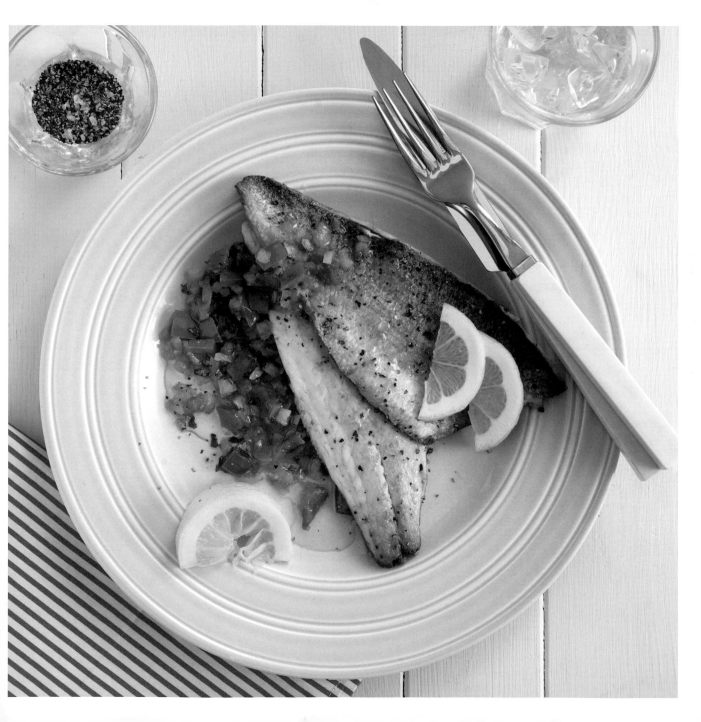

1 tablespoon oil

1 small onion, finely
    chopped

2 teaspoons white wine
    vinegar

⅔ cup fish broth

½ cup heavy cream

Salt and pepper

1 teaspoon lemon juice

1 tablespoon chopped fresh
    chives

1 pound baby spinach
    leaves, washed

2 pats butter, softened

2 lemon sole or flounder
    fillets, skin removed

Fillets of sole with spinach

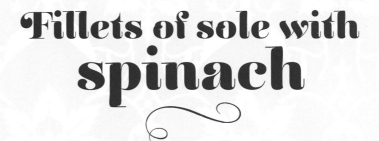

✳ To make the sauce, heat the oil in a saucepan. Add the onion and sauté for 5 minutes, or until soft. Add the vinegar and stir until evaporated. Add the fish broth and reduce by a third. Add the heavy cream and simmer for 2 minutes. Season well with salt and pepper and add the lemon juice and chives. Keep warm.

✳ Preheat the broiler. Wilt the spinach in a large frying pan, drain, and gently squeeze out the excess water. Melt 1 of the pats of butter in the pan. Return the spinach to the pan and season with salt and pepper. Sauté for 1 to 2 minutes, until heated through.

✳ While the spinach is cooking, arrange the fish on a greased baking sheet. Spread the remaining 1 pat of butter over the fillets and season well with salt and pepper. Broil for 5 to 6 minutes, until the fish is firm and opaque. Arrange the spinach on two plates, top with the fish, and pour on the sauce.

The roasted red pepper, shallot, and tomato sauce is delicious with fish. This recipe uses roasted cod, but the sauce also complements other fish, such as branzino fillets.

• • •

MAKES 4 PORTIONS
SUITABLE FOR FREEZING

2 red bell peppers
3 tablespoons olive oil
2 shallots, finely chopped
1 clove garlic, crushed
4 ripe tomatoes, peeled, seeded, and chopped
Scant 1 cup vegetable broth
1 teaspoon sugar
Salt and pepper
2 tablespoons butter, softened
4 cod fillets, skin removed
2 teaspoons lemon juice

Roast cod
with roasted red pepper and tomato sauce

✳ Preheat the oven to 400°F.

✳ Bake the red bell peppers, turning occasionally, until browned, about 30 minutes. Place in a plastic bag, let cool, and remove the skins. Core, seed, and coarsely chop.

✳ Heat 1 tablespoon olive oil and sauté the shallots until softened but not browned. Add the garlic and sauté for 30 seconds. Add the tomatoes and cook for 5 minutes, or until soft. Add the peppers, broth, and sugar and cook for 5 minutes. Transfer the mixture to a blender and puree. Return to the pan and season to taste with salt and pepper. Whisk in the butter.

✳ Season the fish with a little salt and pepper. Line a baking pan with foil and brush the foil with 1 tablespoon of the remaining oil. Place the fish on the foil and brush with the remaining 1 tablespoon oil. Sprinkle with the lemon juice, then bake for 15 minutes. Serve with the sauce poured on top.

Cod is very low in fat, which makes it easy to digest. This tomato and caper sauce makes it even more delicious. This dish is also good served on a bed of spinach, which is an excellent nutrient source during pregnancy.

• • •

Cod with tomato and caper sauce

MAKES 2 PORTIONS

Two 5-ounce cod fillets,
  skin removed
5 tablespoons olive oil
Salt and pepper
Juice of half a small lemon
2 tablespoons nonpareil
  capers
2 tomatoes, peeled, seeded,
  and chopped
1 tablespoon finely chopped
  fresh parsley
Handful of caperberries,
  to serve (optional)

✶ Preheat the oven to 400°F.

✶ Put the cod on a baking sheet lined with parchment paper. Drizzle with 1 tablespoon of the olive oil and season with salt and pepper. Bake for 8 to 10 minutes, until just cooked through.

✶ While the fish is cooking, pour the remaining 4 tablespoons of oil into a saucepan. Add the lemon juice. Gently warm through, then add the capers and tomatoes. Pour the sauce over the cod, then sprinkle with the parsley. Serve with a few caperberries, if using.

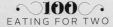

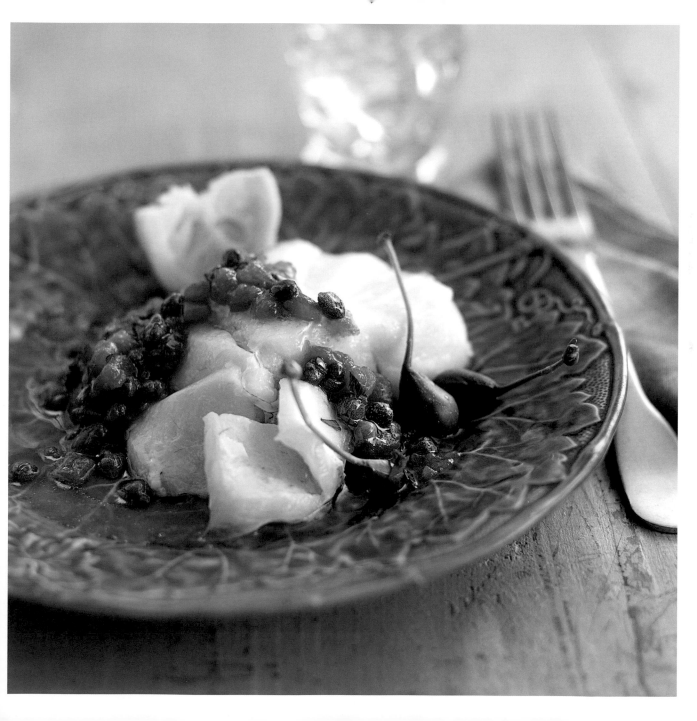

This Asian-style recipe takes only minutes to prepare.

• • •

MAKES 2 PORTIONS

2 tablespoons mirin
¼ cup sweet chili sauce
2 tablespoons honey
4 teaspoons soy sauce
1 teaspoon rice vinegar
4 teaspoons canola oil
1 clove garlic, crushed
½ teaspoon grated fresh ginger
1 large carrot, cut into
   matchsticks
½ red bell pepper, cut into
   matchsticks
4 ears baby corn, halved
   lengthwise
1 zucchini, cut into matchsticks
   or ribbons
2 large scallions, thinly sliced
3 ounces fine egg (chow mein)
   noodles, cooked following
   the package instructions
Two 1-inch-thick tuna steaks
   (about 4 ounces each)

Sticky tuna and fine noodles

✴ Mix together the mirin, 2 tablespoons of the sweet chili sauce, the honey, 1 teaspoon of the soy sauce, and the vinegar and set aside.

✴ Heat 3 teaspoons of the oil in a wok, add the garlic and ginger, and let sizzle for 30 seconds; add the carrot, red bell pepper, and baby corn and stir-fry for 2 minutes. Add the zucchini and scallions and stir-fry for 1 minute. Add the noodles, the remaining 3 teaspoons soy sauce, and the remaining 2 tablespoons sweet chili sauce and stir-fry for 2 minutes. Set the wok aside while you cook the tuna.

✴ To cook the tuna, put the remaining teaspoon oil in a nonstick frying pan and place over high heat until hot. Add the tuna and cook for about 1½ minutes on each side, or until cooked through, then transfer to a plate.

✴ Reduce the heat and add the mirin mix to the pan. Boil for 1 to 2 minutes, until syrupy. Remove from the heat and let cool slightly, then return the tuna to the pan and turn to coat in the sauce.

✴ Divide the noodle mixture between plates. Serve with the tuna (sliced, if desired) and spoon on the sauce from the pan.

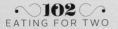

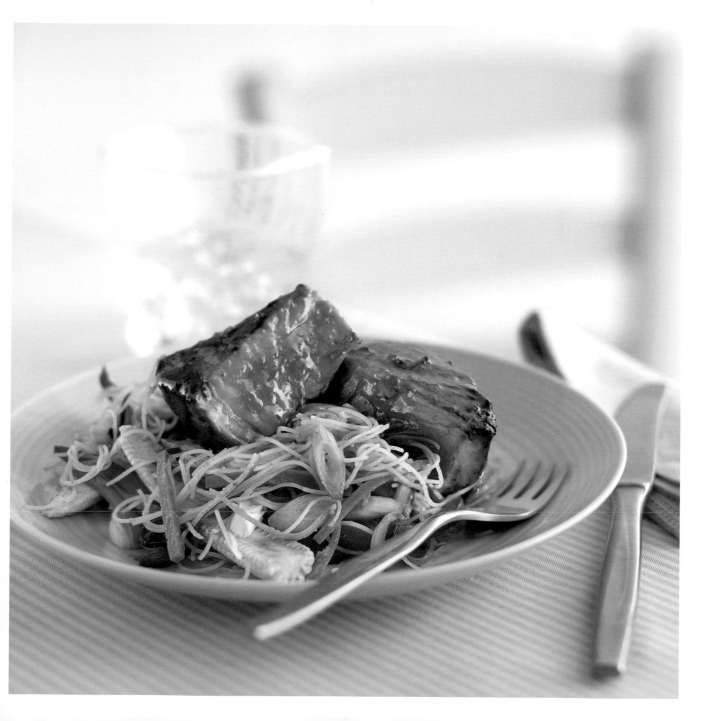

1 tablespoon plus 1 pat of
butter
1 onion, finely diced
5 cups (loosely packed) baby
spinach, washed
Salt and pepper
2 tablespoons all-purpose
flour
Scant 1 cup milk
⅓ cup grated Parmesan
cheese
1 teaspoon Dijon mustard
Two 5-ounce haddock or cod
fillets, skin removed
2 tablespoons fresh bread
crumbs
⅓ cup grated Gruyère cheese
½ teaspoon paprika

Haddock
Florentine

✷ RICH IN IRON ✷

✷ Preheat the oven to 400°F.

✷ Melt the pat of butter in a saucepan. Add the onion and
sauté for 5 minutes, or until soft. Heat the spinach in a frying pan until wilted, then drain; add to the onion. Season
well with salt and pepper.

✷ To make the sauce, melt the tablespoon of butter in a
saucepan. Add the flour and mix together over the heat.
Blend in the milk gradually, stirring until thickened.
Season with salt and pepper and add the Parmesan and
mustard. Add 2 tablespoons of the sauce to the spinach.

✷ On a cutting board, slice each haddock fillet in half cross-
wise so that you have four pieces. Spoon the spinach on top
of two pieces of the haddock, then put the other two pieces
on top of the spinach, so they are sandwiched together.

✷ Place in a shallow ovenproof dish. Pour in the remaining
sauce and sprinkle with the bread crumbs, Gruyère, and
paprika.

✷ Bake for 20 to 25 minutes, until golden and bubbling.
Let stand for 5 minutes before serving.

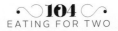

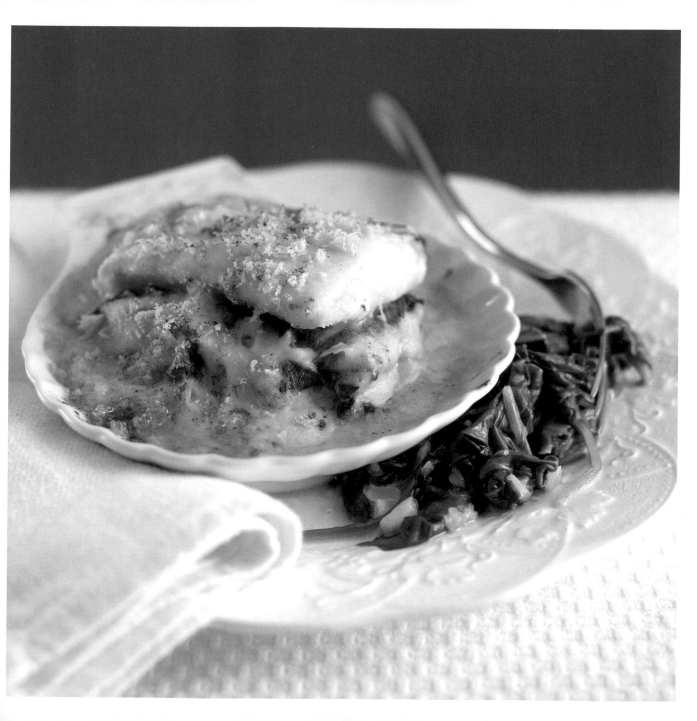

As summer approaches, it is good to eat tasty, light meals like this delicious salad with a Japanese-style dressing. Many of the prepared salads that you can buy lack flavor, and nothing tastes as good as a fresh salad you've made yourself. The crunchy texture of the diced cucumber and red bell pepper complements the moist salmon and rice.

• • •

MAKES 4 PORTIONS

12 ounces salmon fillet, skin removed
Pat of butter
1 cup long-grain rice
1⅔ cups frozen peas
1 red bell pepper, finely diced
½ cucumber, peeled, seeded, and diced
1 small bunch scallions, thinly sliced
2 tablespoons chopped fresh Italian parsley
2 tablespoons chopped fresh dill
2 tablespoons chopped fresh chives
2 tablespoons olive oil
3 tablespoons rice vinegar
2 teaspoons honey
Salt and pepper

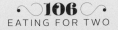
Salmon
and rice salad

✳ Preheat the oven to 350°F.

✳ Put the salmon fillet on a piece of foil on a baking sheet. Top with the butter. Fold the foil over and around the salmon to form a package, then fold and seal the edges. Cook in the oven for 15 minutes, or until the flesh is cooked through. Remove from the oven and let cool. (Alternatively, cut the salmon into chunks and poach in a saucepan of fish broth over low heat for about 7 minutes, or until the flesh flakes easily with a fork.)

✳ Cook the rice in boiling salted water following the package instructions. Add the peas to the pan 4 minutes before the end of the cooking time. Drain in a strainer and refresh under running water. Set aside.

✳ Place all the remaining ingredients except the salt and pepper in a large bowl. Add the cooked rice and peas, then flake in the cooled salmon and any cooking juices from the foil. Season well with salt and pepper, then cover and refrigerate for 30 minutes before serving.

Orzo is pasta that looks like rice. If you can't find it, then you could use any small pasta shapes, such as mini pasta shells.

• • •

MAKES 4 PORTIONS

8 ounces orzo pasta
1 bunch of scallions, sliced
3 tablespoons drained canned corn
One 6-ounce can tuna in oil, drained
1 large tomato, seeded and diced
¼ cucumber, peeled, seeded, and diced
Salt and pepper
2 tablespoons crème fraîche or reduced-fat sour cream
2 tablespoons light mayonnaise
1½ tablespoons ketchup
1½ teaspoons lemon juice
1 teaspoon rice vinegar

Tuna orzo salad

✻ Cook the orzo following the package instructions, drain, and refresh under running water. Mix with the scallions, corn, tuna, tomato, and cucumber. Season to taste with salt and pepper. Mix the crème fraîche, mayonnaise, ketchup, lemon juice, and vinegar together and pour over the pasta. Mix well.

These fish cakes are deliciously moist, as I don't cook the fish first. Cooking potatoes in their skins before using prevents them from becoming too mushy.

• • •

MAKES 8 FISH CAKES
SUITABLE FOR FREEZING

1 large (about 9 ounces) baked potato, skin removed, cut into chunks
5 tablespoons mayonnaise
3½ tablespoons sweet chili sauce
1 teaspoon lemon juice
3 tablespoons thinly sliced scallion
⅓ cup grated Cheddar cheese
2 tablespoons ketchup
8 ounces salmon fillet, skin removed, cut into small cubes
1 cup fresh bread crumbs
Salt and pepper
1 heaping cup dried bread crumbs, for coating
3 to 4 tablespoons canola oil

Salmon fish cakes

✳ Mix the potato chunks with 2 tablespoons of the mayonnaise, 1½ tablespoons of the sweet chili sauce, the lemon juice, scallion, Cheddar, and ketchup and coarsely mash, using a potato masher. Mix in the salmon cubes and fresh bread crumbs and season to taste with salt and pepper.

✳ Using your hands, form the mixture into 8 fish cakes. Coat with the dried bread crumbs. Heat the oil in a large frying pan and sauté the cakes for about 5 minutes, turning halfway through, or until golden on both sides and the salmon is cooked through.

✳ To make a dip, simply mix together the remaining 3 tablespoons mayonnaise and 2 tablespoons sweet chili sauce.

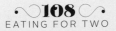

Salmon provides a brain-building dose of omega-3 oils, as well as valuable protein—but watch your intake while pregnant. It's advised that you don't consume more than two portions of oily fish a week.

• • •

MAKES 2 PORTIONS

2 heaping tablespoons low-fat cream cheese

3 tablespoons chopped fresh chives

5 teaspoons chopped fresh basil

2 teaspoons chopped fresh dill

1 tablespoon lemon juice

Salt and pepper

Two 4-ounce salmon fillets, skin removed

3 tablespoons fine fresh bread crumbs

3 tablespoons grated Parmesan cheese

2 tomatoes, seeded and chopped

2 scallions, chopped

1 tablespoon olive oil

2 tablespoons white wine vinegar

Salmon fillets with tomato salsa

✶ RICH IN OMEGA-3 OILS ✶

✶ Preheat the oven to 400°F.

✶ To make the topping, combine the cream cheese, 2 tablespoons of the chives, 2 teaspoons of the basil, the dill, and lemon juice and season to taste with salt and pepper.

✶ Spread the mixture over the top of each piece of fish, covering the whole fillet. Place on a baking sheet. Mix the bread crumbs, Parmesan, and the remaining 1 tablespoon chives together. Sprinkle over the fillets. Bake for 12 to 15 minutes, until the salmon is cooked through and the topping is lightly golden brown. If the topping is a little pale, you can quickly brown it under a hot broiler to crisp it.

✶ To make the salsa, mix together the tomatoes, scallions, olive oil, vinegar, and the remaining 1 tablespoon basil. Season with salt and pepper and serve with the salmon.

This salad will serve up a range of nutrients and valuable fiber. And the ginger can help with morning sickness.

• • •

MAKES 4 PORTIONS

2 tablespoons soy sauce
¼ cup olive oil
1 teaspoon sweet chili sauce
½ teaspoon grated fresh ginger
1 clove garlic, crushed
Two 8-ounce salmon fillets, skin removed
2 slices white bread
1 small heart of romaine lettuce, coarsely chopped
½ red bell pepper, seeded and diced
3 tablespoons drained canned corn
1 avocado, peeled and sliced
½ cup shaved Parmesan cheese
3 tablespoons light mayonnaise
2 teaspoons lemon juice
1 teaspoon rice vinegar
A few drops of Worcestershire sauce
1 tablespoon water
Pinch of sugar

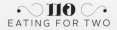
Salmon salad

✳ Preheat the oven to 400°F.

✳ Mix together the soy sauce, 2 tablespoons of the oil, the chili sauce, ginger, and garlic in a shallow dish. Add the salmon and marinate for 30 minutes in the fridge.

✳ To make croutons, cut the bread into cubes and toss in the remaining 2 tablespoons oil. Place on a baking sheet and toast for 15 minutes, until golden and crisp.

✳ Heat an ovenproof frying pan until hot. Cook the salmon for 1 minute on each side. Pour in the marinade, then transfer to the oven. Bake for 10 minutes, or until cooked through. Let cool.

✳ Arrange the lettuce on a platter. Scatter with the diced pepper, corn, and avocado. Add the croutons.

✳ Cut the salmon into thick slices and arrange on the salad. Scatter with the Parmesan shavings.

✳ Combine the mayonnaise, lemon juice, vinegar, Worcestershire sauce, water, and sugar. Drizzle on the salad.

8 ounces penne
2 tablespoons olive oil
1 red onion, sliced
4 plum tomatoes, quartered, seeded, and coarsely chopped
One 6-ounce can tuna in oil, drained
½ cup oven-roasted tomatoes or ¼ cup oil-packed sun-dried tomatoes, drained and chopped
1 teaspoon balsamic vinegar
Handful of basil leaves, torn into pieces
Salt and pepper

Penne with tuna, tomato, and red onion

✳ Cook the penne following the package instructions. Drain.

✳ Meanwhile, heat the oil in a frying pan, add the onion, and cook, stirring occasionally, for about 6 minutes, or until softened. Stir in the fresh tomatoes and cook for 2 to 3 minutes, until beginning to soften. Add the tuna, oven-roasted or sun-dried tomatoes, balsamic vinegar, basil, salt and pepper to taste and heat for 1 minute before stirring into the pasta.

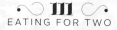

Both basmati rice and peas are low-GI foods— carbohydrates that are released slowly and thus fuel the body for longer.

• • •

MAKES 4 PORTIONS
SUITABLE FOR FREEZING

1 cup basmati rice
1¼ cups frozen peas
1 pound salmon fillet, skin removed
¼ cup water
2 tablespoons lemon juice
Salt and pepper
1 tablespoon canola oil
1 large onion, thinly sliced
2 tablespoons mild korma curry paste (such as Patak's)
2 tablespoons chopped fresh cilantro (optional)
¼ cup sliced almonds, toasted (optional)

Salmon and pea kedgeree

✳ Cook the rice following the package instructions. Add the peas for the last few minutes of cooking. Drain, spread out on a plate, and let cool slightly.

✳ Put the salmon in a microwavable dish with the water and 1 tablespoon of the lemon juice, plus a little salt and pepper. Cover, leaving a steam vent, and cook for 2 to 4 minutes on high, or until just cooked through. Alternatively, you can poach the salmon in a frying pan in fish broth for about 8 to 10 minutes. Transfer the salmon to a plate and flake into chunks. Reserve the cooking liquid.

✳ Heat the oil in a large frying pan or wok and sauté the onion for 8 to 10 minutes, until golden. Stir in the curry paste and cook for 1 minute, then remove from the heat and stir in the rice and peas. Season with salt and pepper and stir in the remaining 1 tablespoon lemon juice, and 1 tablespoon of the salmon cooking liquid. Gently fold in the fish.

✳ To serve, stir in the chopped cilantro and sprinkle with the toasted sliced almonds, if using.

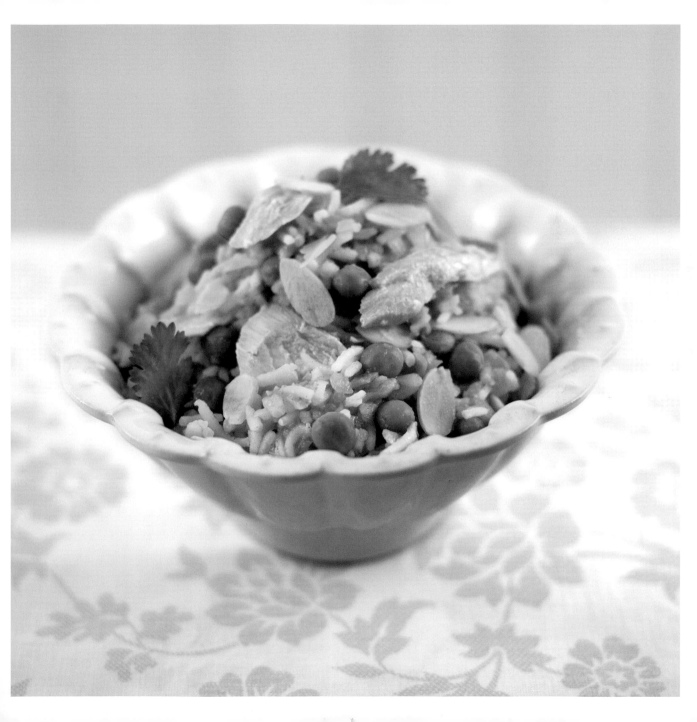

MAKES 4 PORTIONS
SUITABLE FOR FREEZING

12 ounces potatoes, peeled
and diced
3 scallions, chopped
1 heaping tablespoon
capers, chopped
½ cup grated sharp Cheddar
cheese
One 6-ounce can tuna,
drained
Juice of half a lemon
Salt and pepper
All-purpose flour for dusting
1 egg, beaten
1 cup Japanese-style (panko)
bread crumbs
Olive oil and butter, for
frying

Tuna and caper fish cakes

✳ Put the potatoes into cold salted water. Bring to a boil, and once cooked, drain and mash.

✳ Put the scallions, capers, Cheddar, tuna, and lemon juice in a bowl. Add the mashed potatoes, season well with salt and pepper, and mix together. Shape into 4 large fish cakes. Dust lightly with flour, then dip in the beaten egg, and coat with the bread crumbs.

✳ Heat a little oil and a pat of butter in a frying pan. Fry the fish cakes until golden, about 5 minutes on each side.

✳ Serve with a green salad and mayonnaise.

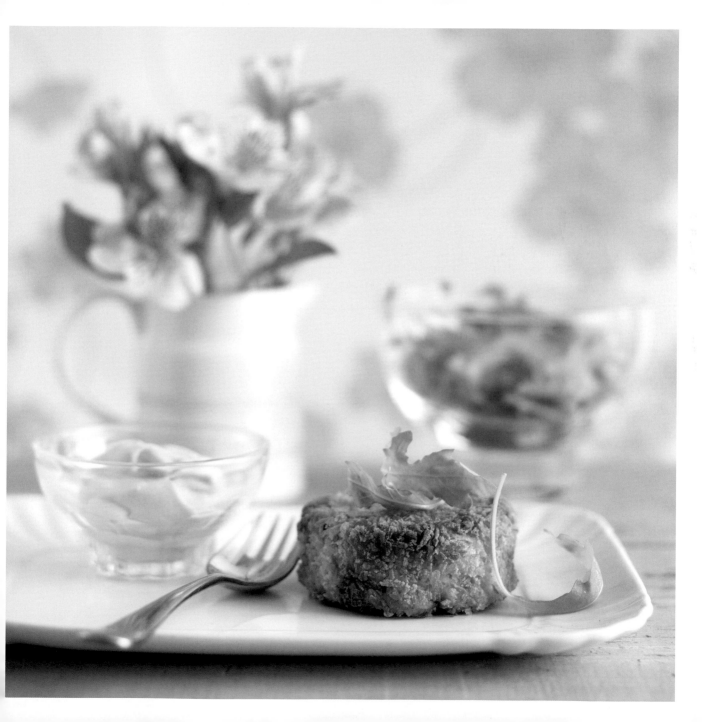

2 large gray sole fillets
   (about 4 ounces each),
   skin removed
Salt and pepper
¼ cup all-purpose flour
1 egg, beaten
2 cups Japanese-style
   (panko) bread crumbs or
   fine dried bread crumbs
1 tablespoon canola oil
Juice of half a lemon

Tartar Sauce
¼ cup mayonnaise
2 tablespoons finely
   chopped cornichons
1 scallion, chopped
1 tablespoon capers,
   chopped
1 teaspoon lemon juice
Salt and pepper

Gray
sole goujons with tartar sauce

✳ Slice each fillet lengthwise into 3 or 4 pieces. Season with salt and pepper, then dust with the flour. Dip the goujons in the egg, then coat with the bread crumbs. Heat the oil in a frying pan. Fry the goujons for 1½ to 2 minutes on each side, until golden and crisp and the fish is cooked through. Drain on paper towels, season with salt and pepper, and squeeze on the lemon juice.

✳ To make the sauce, mix together the mayonnaise, cornichons, scallion, capers, and 1 teaspoon lemon juice. Season with salt and pepper. Serve with the goujons.

A delicious low-fat way to prepare fish in under 15 minutes.

• • •

MAKES 4 PORTIONS

4 small branzino fillets, skin on
Salt and pepper
2 tablespoons canola oil
¾-inch piece of fresh ginger, julienned
2 cloves garlic, thinly sliced
2 tablespoons soy sauce
2 tablespoons mirin
1 bunch of scallions, shredded

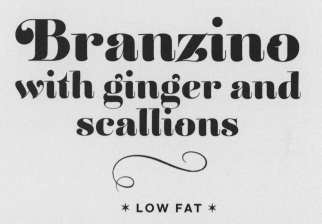

Branzino
with ginger and scallions

✳ **LOW FAT** ✳

✳ Season the fish with salt and pepper and slash the skin.

✳ Heat 1 tablespoon of the oil in a large frying pan and fry the fish, skin side down, for 3 to 4 minutes, until the skin is crispy. Flip and fry on the other side for 1 minute. Remove from the pan and keep warm.

✳ Heat the remaining 1 tablespoon oil. Fry the ginger and garlic for 1 minute, then add the soy sauce, mirin, and scallions and cook briefly. Return the fish to the pan, spoon the sauce over the fish, and heat through.

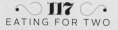

You can freeze the fish once it is coated but before it is cooked.

• • •

MAKES 2 PORTIONS

2 medium sweet potatoes, scrubbed
2 tablespoons olive oil
4 or 5 slices whole wheat bread, crusts removed
¼ cup grated Parmesan cheese
2 tablespoons coarsely chopped fresh chives
Pinch of paprika
Salt and pepper
¼ cup all-purpose flour
1 egg
1 teaspoon water
Skinless fillets of flounder or gray sole from 2 small fish
Canola oil

Dip
3 tablespoons mayonnaise (reduced-fat variety is fine)
2 tablespoons Greek yogurt
2 tablespoons lemon juice
1 tablespoon snipped fresh chives

New-style
fish and chips

✳ Preheat the oven to 400°F.

✳ Cut the potatoes into wedges and put in a bowl. Toss with the olive oil and spread out on 2 baking sheets. Bake for 35 to 40 minutes, turning every 10 minutes, until browned at the edges. Watch carefully toward the end of the cooking time.

✳ Put the bread, Parmesan, chives, and paprika in a food processor and whiz until you make bread crumbs. Season with salt and pepper and spread out on a plate. Put the flour on another plate and season with salt and pepper. Whisk the egg with the water in a shallow bowl.

✳ Dust the fish with the flour, dip in the egg, and roll in the crumbs to coat. Put on a tray. Heat a thin layer of canola oil in a large frying pan and fry the fish over medium heat for 2 to 3 minutes on each side, until golden and cooked through (you may need to do this in two batches).

✳ Blot on paper towels before serving with the potatoes.

✳ To make the dip, simply whisk together the mayonnaise, yogurt, lemon juice, and chives.

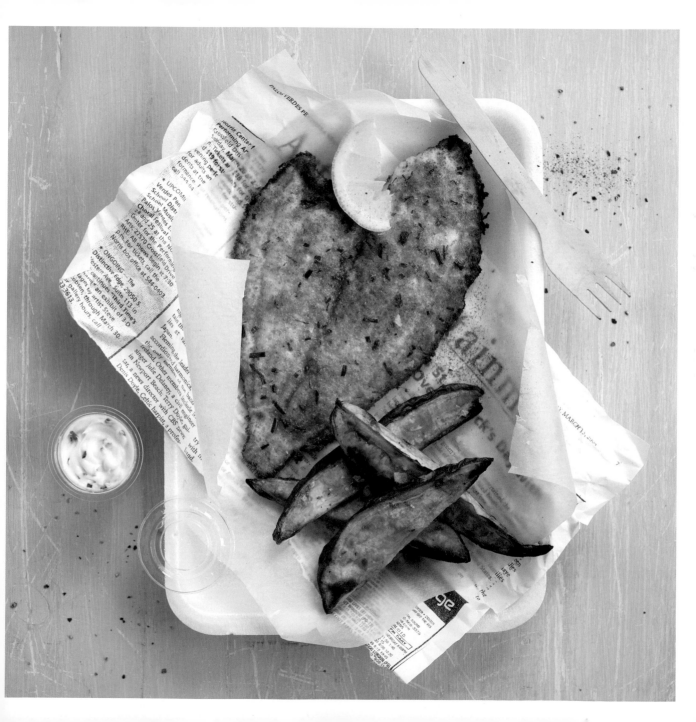

4: The Third Trimester

The Third Trimester: A time for growth

As you'll be able to feel, your baby grows most rapidly in the third trimester. Her weight will skyrocket during this time, from around just under 2 pounds to from 6 to 9 pounds—keep in mind that healthy babies come in a range of sizes. As hard as it is to believe if this is your first pregnancy, by the end of the trimester you'll have a real, fully grown baby squirming around inside you.

You'll continue to grow, too. By the end of the trimester you'll probably have reached the weight gain recommended for pregnancy. Some women find that their weight gain slows a little toward the end of the pregnancy. As well as nourishing your baby during this time, it's a priority to make sure you're eating well enough to keep your own nutritional stores topped up. Your body will need all the preparation possible for the birth, and for bodily repair and breast-feeding afterward.

The nutritional issues that are common during this trimester may also have occurred earlier in the pregnancy. However, the increased rate of your baby's growth means that problems such as heartburn and anemia become more frequent. Another less medical problem of this trimester is what I call "pregnancy burnout"—when you feel fed up with pregnancy and all its stress and guidelines. Read on in this chapter for advice on all these issues.

This brings us to after the pregnancy. While it may be (almost) the last thing on your mind at the moment, there will come a time when you will no longer be pregnant! You have heard it before, but it's hard to believe how busy you'll be at home with a new baby. A few hours spent preparing your freezer as well as your nursery will seem like time well spent in a few months when you're trying to feed yourself as well as your baby.

Nutrition priorities during the third trimester

There are so many reasons why it's important to eat well in the third trimester—supporting your baby's rocketing growth rate, supporting your own body's rocketing growth rate, maximizing your baby's nutritional stores for after the birth (particularly iron), and maximizing your own stores for the stresses of labor, and for recovery and breast-feeding afterward. Your calorie requirements actually increase at this point: an extra 200 calories per day. To get some idea how much food this translates to, have a look at page 122. Other nutrients that are especially important at this time include calcium, because the baby's developing bones are increasingly using the calcium in your diet, and iron, to prevent anemia and to provide ample amounts to build the baby's stores. Later in this chapter (page 122) there's information on increasing iron intake. One last nutrient to pay special attention to at this time is omega-3 fats. They make up a proportion of your baby's growing brain, nerves, and eyes, and studies have found an association between a mother's intake of omega-3s

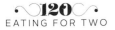

and her child's IQ. You might like to review the guidelines on pages 12 and 27 for the sources of omega-3s and limits on fish that contain them.

At the same time as your requirements increase, you may feel a change from the hunger of the second trimester, and find it increasingly difficult to fit enough food in during the third trimester. As your baby grows larger, she leaves less room for the rest of what's inside you, including your stomach. Many women also experience digestive problems such as heartburn and constipation (see page 72). These problems can make it difficult to eat the same size meals you are used to. It may be some consolation that you'll have a little more space once your baby moves lower into your pelvis in the last weeks of pregnancy.

If you're concerned that you're not fitting in all the foods your body requires, keep a food diary for a few days and go through the food groups (see chapter 1) to work out if you're missing anything. If so, here are a few ideas to help you fit the food in:

* Eat smaller meals but plan regular, larger snacks. The snacks don't have to be "snacky" food and can be mini meals such as a sandwich or cereal.
* Remember that drinks will fill you up as well as food. To avoid becoming too full, try to drink between, rather than with, meals.
* Skip sugary and fatty foods. Your priority is for maximum nutrition. Foods high in sugar or fat will fill you up, but probably not supply large amounts of other nutrients.
* You could try "drinking" some of the foods you're having trouble fitting in, choosing instead reduced-fat milk drinks, fruit juices and smoothies, and vegetable juices and soups (though look out for those with added salt).

If you still feel your intake may not be meeting your needs, talk to your ob-gyn and consider taking a pregnancy multivitamin and mineral supplement if you're not on one already.

You and your baby during the third trimester

You

If this is your first baby, she will probably drop lower into your pelvis by about 38 weeks. This will ease the pressure on your stomach and lungs but will increase the weight resting on your bladder.

• • •

Keep up your supply of omega-3 fats for your baby's brain and visual development —almost three-quarters of her brain develops in the last trimester.

• • •

Aim for a weight gain of just under 1 pound a week during these three months. Aim to gain a little more if you started the pregnancy underweight, and a little less if you were overweight.

Your baby

Your baby's weight gain is rapid in this trimester—part of this is fat stores she is laying down under her skin.

• • •

At the end of 32 weeks your baby is beginning to store minerals such as iron, calcium, and phosphorus— these all come from your diet. In addition, extra calcium is needed as your baby's bones and teeth develop. Your baby will also be laying down a reserve of iron for the first 6 months of life, when her iron intake will be low.

• • •

At birth your baby is likely to weigh between 6 and 9 pounds.

Ten 200-calorie foods

* Small handful of almonds, small handful of cranberries, and 1 teaspoon of sunflower seeds
* 3 rice cakes spread with reduced-fat garlic-and-herb cream cheese and topped with 6 cherry tomatoes
* 1 cup low-fat fruit yogurt and 1 cup fruit salad
* A hard-boiled egg with 2 slices of whole wheat toast and butter or margarine
* Small baked potato with 3 tablespoons grated reduced-fat cheese
* 1 cup hot chocolate made with reduced-fat milk
* 2 rye crispbreads with 3 tablespoons drained canned tuna and 1 tablespoon reduced-fat mayonnaise
* 3 tablespoons hummus with 6 carrot sticks and 3 breadsticks
* Smoothie made with 1 small banana, ¾ cup plain low-fat yogurt, and 1 teaspoon honey
* Small portion lentil soup and a whole wheat cracker

Nutritional issues

Anemia

Iron-deficiency anemia is a common problem during pregnancy, despite our bodies' clever mechanism of absorbing more iron than usual during this time. This is partly because a pregnant woman's iron requirement is dramatically higher than that of other women—extra is required to form the baby's red blood cells and to make more for the mother so she can carry oxygen for her baby as well as herself. While the main symptom of anemia is tiredness (even more than the usual pregnancy exhaustion), consequences can be serious. For example, left untreated, anemia is linked with premature labor and low birth weight in babies, and severe cases can cause an irregular heartbeat in the mother.

You are likely to be tested for iron-deficiency anemia during your pregnancy. If you are at risk or are anemic, follow the guidelines below to increase your iron intake. Do note that the type of iron found in meat, fish, and poultry is more easily absorbed than that found in plant foods. However, absorption of the iron from plant foods can be boosted by eating them with meat or with foods rich in vitamin C. See the list below for ideas on how to do this. You can also find more information on iron in Pregnancy Supernutrients, on page 16.

Sometimes even the best iron-rich diet isn't enough and you may find that iron supplements are required. Some people find that iron supplements play havoc with their bowels. If you're having problems, you may want to check out the information on constipation on page 72. You could also ask your pharmacist or ob-gyn to suggest a different iron supplement.

Top 10 ways to boost iron levels
* Red meats such as beef and lamb are a great, easily absorbed source of iron.
* Dark chicken meat, such as the thighs.
* Oil-rich fish, such as salmon, tuna, sardines, and mackerel, contain easily absorbed iron.
* Fortified breakfast cereal is high in iron—check the label to see if iron has been added.
* Fortified bread is a convenient source of iron.
* Green leafy vegetables, including kale, broccoli, bok choy, and watercress, contain valuable

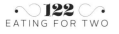

amounts of iron. Legumes, such as dried beans, split peas, lentils, and chickpeas, are another plant source of iron.

* Dried fruits such as apricots, figs, prunes, and raisins are an iron-rich way to snack.
* Nuts and seeds, including pumpkin and sunflower seeds, Brazil nuts, and walnuts, are also a source of iron. Try them sprinkled on breakfast cereal or desserts.
* Adding a source of vitamin C to vegetable sources of iron will boost their absorption. Foods rich in vitamin C include citrus fruits and juices, melon, berries, tomatoes, and peppers. Alternatively, an animal source such as red meat will help the absorption of iron from plant foods. For example, gain an iron boost by drinking orange juice with peanut butter on toast or fortified breakfast cereal, enjoy a beef and leafy green vegetable stir-fry, or lunch on lentil soup with a tomato salad on the side.
* Avoid drinking tea or coffee with meals, as they may block absorption of some of the iron. Calcium may also have this effect, so try to consume milk drinks and other dairy foods such as yogurt and pudding at snack times rather than with main meals if your iron levels are low. Note that eggs are another food that blocks iron absorption.

Heartburn

This painful condition can occur throughout pregnancy, but never more so than during the third trimester. Throughout pregnancy the muscle that prevents acidic gastric juices from rising out of the

Pregnancy Myth buster: I should eat liver to boost my iron levels

While it's true that liver is a great source of easily absorbed iron, it's also high in vitamin A. During pregnancy, high levels of vitamin A have been associated with damage to unborn babies. For this reason, pregnant women should avoid eating liver and foods made from it, such as pâté and liverwurst. Check out the ideas on page 122 for boosting iron levels with alternative iron-rich foods.

stomach into the esophagus (the tube that takes food to your stomach) doesn't work as well due to hormones. In the third trimester the pressure of your baby on the stomach also causes the juices to rise up—there's just not a lot of room for your baby and your bodily organs. While there are antacids to reduce the acidity ("burn") of the stomach juices, what and when you eat and drink can also make a huge difference.

Here are some tips to prevent (or at least reduce) heartburn:

* If your stomach doesn't get too full, heartburn is less likely. In practice you can do this by eating smaller main meals with more substantial snacks.
* Fluids as well as food will fill your stomach, so just sip a small amount with food and have most of your drinks an hour or so before or after meals.
* Avoid eating high-fat meals and fried foods, especially at night before bedtime. They tend to stay in your stomach for longer.
* Keep in mind that caffeine-containing drinks

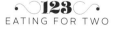

(coffee, tea, and cola), alcohol, and smoking can all further loosen the muscle that stops the stomach contents from rising into the esophagus, thus worsening heartburn. Of course, you'll probably be limiting or avoiding all of these already.

* Sit up straight while eating, and wear loose-fitting clothes.
* Stay upright after eating—gravity helps keep the stomach contents down. Eat your evening meal a few hours before going to bed, and avoid eating or drinking just before taking a nap.
* Some people find raising the head of their bed by a few inches helps. You could put a piece of wood under the bed legs.

You'll hear stories of foods that are reputed to cause heartburn. It's true that certain foods seem to irritate certain people, while other people seem to get away with eating anything. Common culprits are spicy foods and acidic foods such as citrus fruits, tomatoes, and tomato sauces; peppermint; carbonated drinks; and chocolate (possibly because of the small amount of caffeine in it). On the flip side, some women find that the traditional remedy of drinking milk helps. Others find it helps for a little while but then makes the heartburn worse.

Try the suggestions listed above, but if they don't help, speak to your ob-gyn or pharmacist about over-the-counter medications that are suitable during pregnancy.

Pregnancy burnout
This is a time when you may start to feel that enough is enough. You may be tired, achy, and just fed up with being pregnant. The urge to drink alcohol, which happily deserts many women earlier during pregnancy, may return. It can be difficult to continue to follow the myriad guidelines you've been given for just one more day, let alone a few more months. This is the time to focus on your baby, the reason you're going through all this. She may seem almost a figment of your imagination at this point, but, believe me, she'll be here soon enough and all the sacrifices will seem worthwhile.

If you're feeling that you can't face yet another healthy snack, try one of the "naughty (but still nutritious)" treats listed below. Better still, take time out to enjoy it with a pregnant friend so you can have a laugh at all your ailments.

Top 10 naughty (but still nutritious) treats
* Crispbread with Nutella or peanut butter
* Strawberries topped with Greek yogurt (look for the low-fat type) and drizzled with honey
* Chocolate-chip cereal bar
* Banana split: Split a banana and top it with reduced-fat ice cream, chocolate topping, and a sprinkle of chopped nuts
* Small meringue nest with mixed berries and custard or pudding
* Chocolate milk shake
* Scone with reduced-fat cream cheese and jam
* Popcorn seasoned with a little oil or butter and tossed with a flavoring such as grated Parmesan cheese or cinnamon sugar
* A slice of carrot cake or banana bread
* Cheddar cheese melted on a crusty baguette

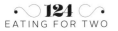

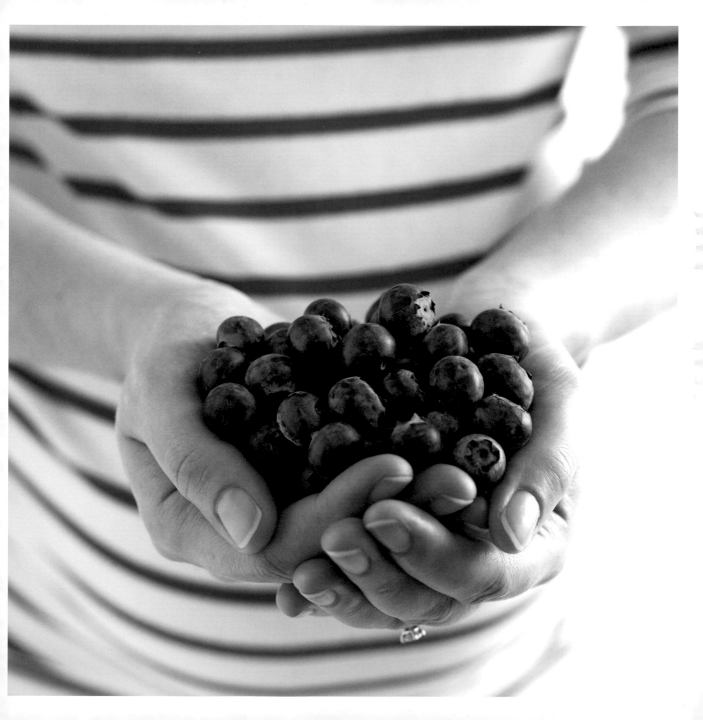

Thinking about the birth

Red raspberry leaf tea

Red raspberry leaf tea may well be the most popular supplement taken during pregnancy, and many women believe it will reduce the duration of labor by toning the muscles of the uterus, thereby increasing the strength of contractions. One study has found an average reduction of nearly ten minutes in the duration of the second (pushing) stage of labor, and reductions in the rate of forceps deliveries. Several have also found no adverse effects on mother or baby. However, other studies have not demonstrated any significant benefit. A recent overall review of the research found that there was little evidence for the benefits of red raspberry leaf tea. And while there is more research into its safety than most other herbs', the reviewers felt that the studies were too small to rule out all effects on unborn babies.

If you are planning to use red raspberry leaf tea, here are a few guidelines: Most important, discuss its use and dosage with your ob-gyn first. Don't start taking it before 32 weeks, and remember that you will need to take it regularly for several weeks before your due date if it's to have any effect. Red raspberry leaf tablets are available if you don't like the taste. Keep in mind that it may not be suitable for you, for example, if you've had complications during a previous labor, are expecting twins or more, or are scheduled to have a cesarean section. Note that there are other herbal teas available containing mixes of herbs for this stage of pregnancy. As always, consult your ob-gyn if you're thinking of taking them, as most substances you take in pass through the placenta to your baby.

Nutrition during labor

Giving birth may be the biggest marathon your body ever tackles. It's impossible to know now if it will last 6 or 16 hours, but having your body in the best state possible will give you a good start. Rest up and try to eat especially well in the weeks before your due date. Many women want to know how many calories are used up in labor, but there's surprisingly little research into it. In any case, the amount would vary widely, depending to a great extent on the length of labor. Interventions such as episiotomies and cesareans also take a toll on the body and require nutrients for repair.

To help maintain energy levels, I suggest you have a light snack every hour or so during early labor. Look for foods that contain fuel in the form of carbohydrates: Grains such as bread, rice, pasta,

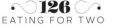

and breakfast cereal; fruit; and yogurt are good choices. If you can't face food, you could sip a drink—maybe fruit juice, flavored water, or a smoothie.

While many women are advised not to eat once at the hospital, a recent review of research into eating and drinking during labor concluded that women should be able to eat and drink as they wish, particularly those at low risk of requiring a general anesthetic. Even if it's not recommended at your hospital, you may be able to negotiate with your ob-gyn about eating or drinking, depending on your stage of labor, so take snacks and some drinks that contain sugar to fuel your body. You may also be incredibly hungry afterward, and there are not a lot of options at most hospitals in the middle of the night, or if you don't have anyone there to fetch you a snack. For this reason, be sure to devote some of your hospital bag (or bags!) to nutritious and portable snacks and drinks. You can look back to the list on page 31 for some ideas.

Thinking ahead to life after the birth

While being 7 to 9 months pregnant, and preparing for the birth, is quite enough to occupy your mind, this is also a time to look ahead to after your baby comes home. You might like to have a quick read through the following chapter and think about freezing some meals for quick and easy dinners when you've had your baby. And if you have your cupboard well stocked with staples such as canned fish, sun-dried tomatoes, pesto and other pasta sauces, pasta, rice, and cans of beans, you'll also be able to put together a meal in minutes. Busy

as you may feel now, you'll probably be more so then.

If you're planning to breast-feed, think ahead to where you might sit, and prepare a "station" where you might keep a bottle of water and snacks. Breast-feeding is thirsty work and you'll spend a lot of time in that spot. A phone, magazine, and TV remote control might come in handy, too.

Top 10 foods to freeze for after the birth
* Your favorite meat sauce for pasta
* Homemade Thai or Indian curry
* Shepherd's pie
* Your favorite soup, maybe lentil and squash, chicken and corn, or potato and leek
* English muffins for breakfast or breast-feeding snacks
* Beef or lentil casserole
* Fruit crisp
* Beef or vegetable lasagna
* Chicken and potato pie (see page 58)
* Fish pie (see page 94)

Can foods induce labor?

The closer you get toward the nine-month mark, the more tales you'll hear of foods that induce labor. A study has shown that more than half of pregnant women in the United States try special foods or other methods to bring on labor. While foods are unlikely to do any harm unless they're specifically to be avoided during pregnancy, keep in mind the issue of dietary balance—any food eaten in excess is likely to prevent you from eating enough of the other foods you require to provide the mix of nutrients your growing baby and you need. Here are a few old favorites:

* Curry and other spicy foods: Some people think that the spices in curry stimulate the nerves of the intestine and, being very close by, might also stimulate the nerves of the uterus. This is purely theoretical; there's no hard evidence, but also no harm in giving it a try if you usually eat spicy food. However, do be aware that it may result in heartburn during pregnancy, and can cause diarrhea in people who aren't used to it. Believe me, this is the last thing you want when going into labor!

* Pineapple: Pineapple contains a substance called bromelain, which some people think will soften the cervix, leading to labor sooner. In fact, there's no evidence for this. There's no harm in eating a few servings of pineapple, but don't consume excessive amounts, as it may lead to mouth ulcers, diarrhea, and being so full that you can't fit in the other foods needed in the diet. Be sure to choose fresh pineapple, because bromelain is destroyed by the canning process.

* Eggplant parmigiana: This recipe doesn't claim any medical reason for inducing labor. However, a restaurant in the state of Georgia claims that most overdue women who eat it there will go into labor in the following days. There's no harm in giving it a try!

Keep in mind that if you're overdue, you have a good chance of going into labor in the next few days, whether you eat these foods or not.

As for any other supplements or herbal remedies (including castor oil, which has been found to be unsafe and can have unpleasant gastrointestinal side effects), the usual advice applies. I suggest you have a discussion with your ob-gyn before taking them.

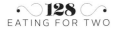

Vegetables

You could make this with or without avocado. If making it without avocado, it will keep for 2 to 3 days. The salad is also good with added raisins.

• • •

MAKES 2 PORTIONS

1⅓ cups quinoa, rinsed
2 cups vegetable broth
6 scallions, thinly sliced
¾ cup roasted unsalted
   cashew nuts
3 tablespoons olive oil
1½ tablespoons lemon juice
Salt and pepper
1 large or 2 small avocados

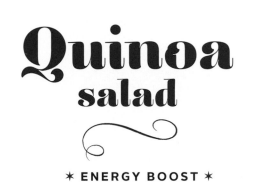

Quinoa
salad

✶ **ENERGY BOOST** ✶

✶ Put the quinoa and broth in a saucepan. Bring to a boil, then reduce the heat and simmer until all the liquid has been absorbed (about 20 minutes). Spread the quinoa out on a plate to cool, then transfer to a bowl.

✶ Stir in the scallions, cashews, oil, and lemon juice and season to taste with salt and pepper. Refrigerate until needed. Just before serving, peel and slice the avocado and lay over the top of the salad.

Tip
Quinoa—pronounced "keen-wha"—is a gluten-free seed that is prepared like a whole grain.
Rich in protein, calcium, and iron, it's a great meat substitute for vegetarians, and is also a good source of fiber.

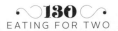

MAKES 2 PORTIONS
SUITABLE FOR FREEZING

Pat of butter
1 onion, chopped
2 leeks, thinly sliced
1 cup peeled and diced
    potatoes
3 cups chicken broth
    (or vegetable broth for
    vegetarians)
1 bay leaf
Pinch of nutmeg
3 to 4 tablespoons heavy
    cream
Salt and pepper
2 tablespoons snipped fresh
    chives

Vichyssoise

✱ Melt the butter in a saucepan. Add the onion and leeks. Gently sauté for 10 minutes, or until soft but without color. Add the potatoes, broth, bay leaf, and nutmeg. Bring to a boil and simmer for about 15 minutes, or until the potatoes are cooked. Remove the bay leaf, then blend until smooth. Pass through a strainer into a bowl. Refrigerate until cold, then add the cream and season to taste with salt and pepper. Add the snipped chives before serving.

MAKES 4 PORTIONS

1¼ pounds very ripe red
    tomatoes, cut into
    quarters
2 tablespoons chopped red
    onion
¼ clove garlic, crushed
1 cup tomato juice
1 tablespoon balsamic
    vinegar
Pinch of sugar

Chilled tomato soup

✱ **LOW FAT** ✱

✱ Put all the ingredients in a food processor and whiz until completely smooth. Pour through a strainer into a bowl. Refrigerate until ready to serve.

1 cup basmati or
   jasmine rice
⅔ cup shelled frozen
   edamame (soy) beans,
   or 3½ cups (8 ounces) if
   unshelled
¼ cup canola oil
4 to 5 tablespoons rice
   vinegar
1 tablespoon sugar
½ teaspoon salt (or to taste)
½ red bell pepper, diced
6 scallions, thinly sliced

Edamame
rice salad

✳ Cook the rice following the package instructions.
Spread out on a plate and let cool for 10 minutes.

✳ Cook the edamame following the package instructions.
Drain and rinse with cold water. Remove the beans from
the shells if necessary. Put in a large bowl and add the rice.

✳ Whisk together the oil, vinegar, sugar, and salt. Stir into
the rice, then add the bell pepper and scallions and stir
again. Refrigerate until ready to serve.

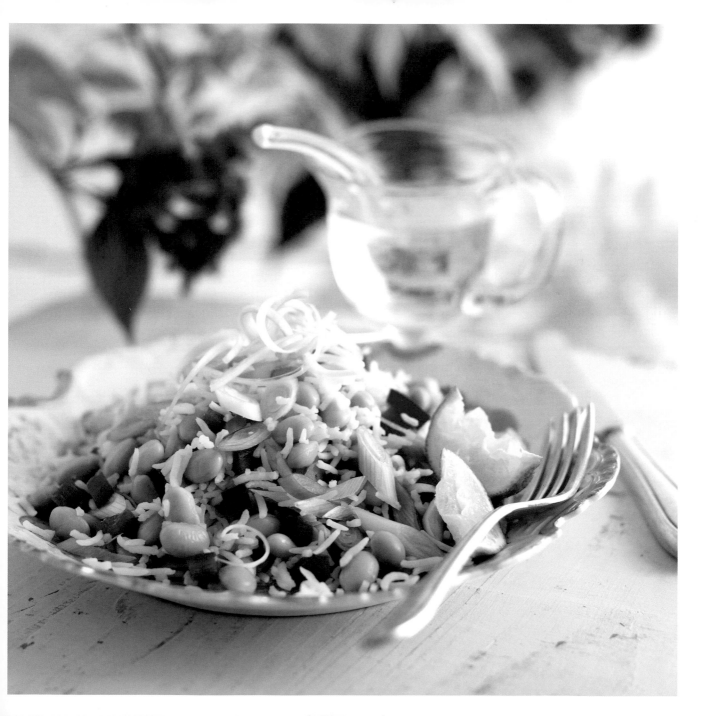

2¼ pounds very red ripe
    tomatoes
½ cucumber, peeled, seeded,
    and coarsely chopped
1 slice white bread, torn into
    pieces
2 tablespoons sherry vinegar
6 tablespoons olive oil
⅔ cup water
Salt and pepper

To serve:
½ cucumber, peeled, seeded,
    and diced
½ red bell pepper, seeded and
    finely diced
2 tablespoons finely chopped
    fresh chives
Olive oil

Gazpacho

✶ Put the tomatoes in a pot of boiling water for 20 seconds, drain, and let cool, then peel off the skins. Slice in half, remove the seeds, and coarsely chop the flesh. Put the tomatoes, cucumber, bread, sherry vinegar, olive oil, and water in a food processor and whiz until very smooth. Pour through a fine strainer into a bowl. Season well with salt and pepper, then refrigerate for 2 hours.

✶ Divide the tomato mixture among four soup bowls and garnish with the cucumber, bell pepper, and chives. Drizzle with a little olive oil before serving.

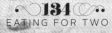

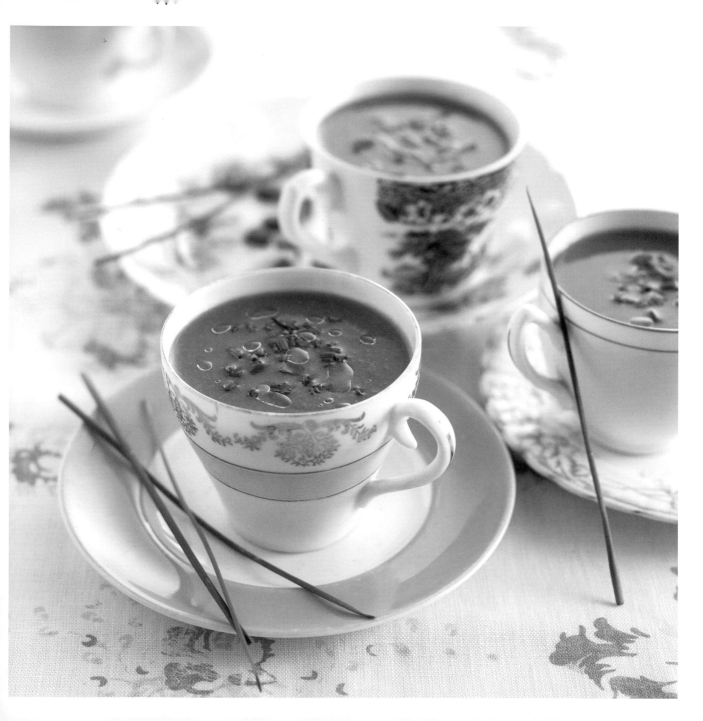

8 ounces fusilli pasta
(or similar)

1 tablespoon butter

1 large leek, white and pale
green parts, rinsed and
thinly sliced

1 clove garlic, crushed

1 cup vegetable broth

1 cup small broccoli florets

⅔ cup frozen peas

1 large tomato, seeded and
diced

6 tablespoons crème fraîche
or heavy cream

3 tablespoons grated
Parmesan cheese

½ cup grated sharp Cheddar
cheese

Salt and pepper

Vegetable fusilli

✴ Cook the pasta following the package instructions.

✴ Meanwhile, melt the butter in a large frying pan or wok
and sauté the leek and garlic for 3 to 4 minutes, until soft.
Add the broth and broccoli and bring to a boil. Reduce the
heat slightly and simmer for 3 to 4 minutes, until the
broccoli is just tender and the broth has reduced to 3 to
4 tablespoons (add a splash of water if the broth evaporates
before the broccoli has cooked). Stir in the remaining
ingredients except the salt and pepper and warm through
until the peas have thawed and the cheeses have melted.

✴ Drain the pasta, reserving a cupful of the cooking water.
Stir the pasta into the sauce in the frying pan. Season to
taste with salt and pepper and add a little of the pasta
cooking water if the pasta is too dry.

Tasty lentil pie

¼ cup olive oil
1 red onion, diced
½ red bell pepper, diced
1 clove garlic, crushed
⅓ cup red lentils
One 14-ounce can diced
 tomatoes
Scant 1 cup vegetable or
 chicken broth
1 teaspoon chopped fresh
 thyme
Salt and pepper
1 to 2 teaspoons mango
 chutney
1 eggplant, thinly sliced
2 tablespoons butter
2 tablespoons all-purpose
 flour
Scant 1 cup milk
3 tablespoons grated
 Parmesan cheese, plus
 extra for the top

✴ Preheat the oven to 400°F.

✴ Heat 1 tablespoon of the oil in a large saucepan.

✴ Add the onion, bell pepper, and garlic. Sauté for 3 to 4 minutes. Add the lentils and coat with the onion mixture. Add the tomatoes, broth, and thyme. Season with salt and pepper, then bring to boil, cover with a lid, and simmer for 20 to 25 minutes, until the lentils are tender. Add the mango chutney, check seasoning, and spoon into a shallow 1½-quart (8 × 8-inch) ovenproof dish.

✴ Heat the remaining 3 tablespoons oil in a frying pan. Fry the eggplant slices on both sides until golden. Arrange over the top of the lentils.

✴ Melt the butter in a saucepan. Add the flour and stir over the heat. Blend in the milk and season with salt and pepper. Bring to a boil, stirring until thickened and smooth. Add the 3 tablespoons Parmesan. Spread over the top of the eggplant and sprinkle with extra Parmesan.

✴ Bake in the oven for 20 to 25 minutes, until golden and bubbling. Let stand for 5 minutes before serving.

1 large tomato
8 ounces fusilli pasta
3 tablespoons butter
4 scallions, thinly sliced
1 clove garlic, crushed
3½ cups (loosely packed)
   baby spinach, coarsely
   chopped
Juice and finely grated zest
   of half a lemon
⅓ cup grated Parmesan
   cheese, plus extra for
   serving
2 tablespoons crème fraîche
   or sour cream
Salt and pepper
2 tablespoons toasted
   pine nuts

Fusilli with spinach and lemon

✳ Bring a large saucepan of salted water to a boil. Cut a cross in the top of the tomato, submerge it in the boiling water for about 30 seconds, and then remove it using a slotted spoon. Hold under cold running water for 10 seconds. Drain.

✳ Add the pasta to the saucepan and cook following the package instructions. Reserve a cupful of the cooking water before draining the pasta. While the pasta cooks, peel, seed, and dice the tomato and set aside.

✳ Melt the butter in a large frying pan and sauté the scallions and garlic for 1 minute. Add the spinach and sauté for 3 to 4 minutes, until it has wilted and any water has evaporated. Stir in 1 tablespoon of the lemon juice and the lemon zest, then add the drained pasta and 1 to 2 table-spoons of the reserved cooking water. Stir together, then remove from the heat and stir in the Parmesan and crème fraîche and season to taste with salt and pepper. Add more water if the pasta is too dry. Transfer to bowls and sprinkle with the pine nuts; serve with extra Parmesan.

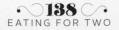

MAKES 6 TO 8 PORTIONS
SUITABLE FOR FREEZING

1 tablespoon canola oil
1 onion, finely chopped
½ medium butternut
squash, peeled, seeded,
and diced
3 tablespoons mild korma
curry paste (such as
Patak's)
1½ cups split red lentils,
rinsed
One 13.5-ounce can
coconut milk
2 cups vegetable broth
Pinch of crushed red pepper
flakes (optional)
Salt and pepper

Mildly spiced lentil and squash soup

✳ Heat the oil in a large saucepan and sauté the onion and squash for 8 to 10 minutes, until the onion is soft. Add the curry paste and cook for 1 minute, then add the lentils, coconut milk, broth, and red pepper flakes (if you would like a bit more heat).

✳ Bring to a boil, then reduce the heat and simmer for 30 to 40 minutes, until the squash and lentils are soft. Let cool slightly, then blend until smooth and season to taste with salt and pepper.

Tip

To reduce the fat content, replace the coconut milk with 1⅔ cups extra broth or use "lite" coconut milk, which contains a lot less fat.

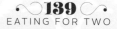

MAKES 3 PORTIONS

Heaping ¾ cup bulgur wheat
1¼ cups cold water
2 teaspoons rice vinegar
Juice of half a lemon
2 tablespoons olive oil
Pinch of sugar
½ small English cucumber,
    diced
1 bunch of scallions, thinly
    sliced
1 small bunch of fresh mint,
    chopped
1 tomato, seeded and
    chopped
2 tablespoons pomegranate
    seeds
Salt and pepper

To serve:
Good-quality store-bought
    hummus and flatbreads
    (optional)

Colorful
tabbouleh

* Put the bulgur wheat in a saucepan and pour in the cold water. Bring to a boil, cover with a lid, and boil for 1 minute. Turn off the heat and let stand (still covered) for 15 minutes, or until all of the liquid has been absorbed.

* Transfer to a bowl. Add the vinegar, lemon juice, olive oil, and sugar. Let cool.

* Add the cucumber, scallions, mint, tomato, pomegranate seeds, and season with salt and pepper to taste; mix well and serve with hummus and flatbreads, if using.

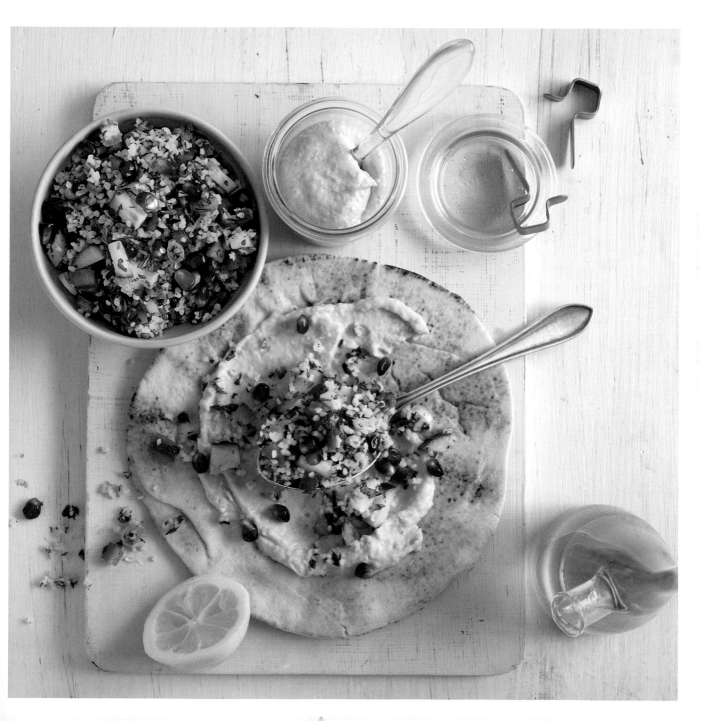

2 cups diced peeled
   butternut squash
3 tablespoons olive oil
Salt and pepper
1 large onion, coarsely
   chopped
2 cloves garlic, crushed
Scant 1 cup risotto rice
3 cups chicken broth
⅓ cup white wine or extra
   chicken broth
¾ cup frozen peas
3 tablespoons grated
   Parmesan cheese
1 teaspoon lemon juice
1 tablespoon chopped fresh
   parsley

Butternut and pea risotto

✳ Preheat the oven to 425°F.

✳ Put the diced butternut squash on a baking sheet. Toss with 1 tablespoon of the oil and season with salt and pepper. Roast in the oven for 25 minutes, or until golden brown. Set aside.

✳ Put the remaining 2 tablespoons oil in a saucepan. Add the onion and garlic and stir over medium heat for 2 to 3 minutes. Add the rice and stir to coat with the mixture. Put the chicken broth in a saucepan, bring to a boil, then add a ladleful of the broth to the rice along with the white wine or additional broth. Stir until absorbed, then continue to add the broth until the rice is cooked. Add the peas after the last of the broth has been added and cook for 5 minutes more. Add the butternut squash, Parmesan, lemon juice, and parsley. Season well with salt and pepper. Serve at once.

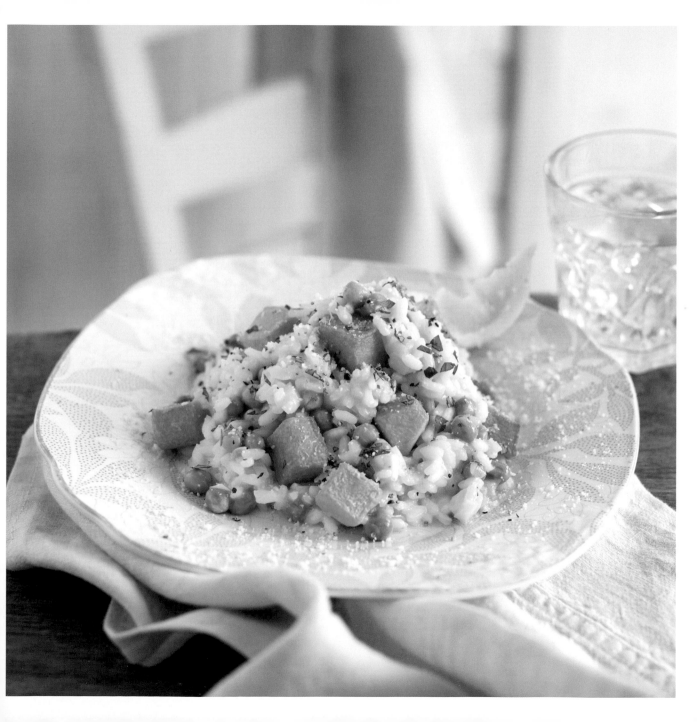

2 tablespoons olive oil
1 large onion, chopped
2 red chiles, seeded
    and diced
2 large cloves garlic, crushed
3½ cups thinly sliced
    cremini mushrooms
⅔ cup drained bottled
    roasted red peppers, sliced
9 cups (loosely packed) baby
    spinach
One 14-ounce can diced
    tomatoes
1 tablespoon tomato paste
Salt and pepper
2 tablespoons chopped fresh
    basil
4 sheets fresh lasagna
    noodles (about 7 ounces)
3 tablespoons butter
¼ cup all-purpose flour
1 cup milk
1 cup crème fraîche or heavy
    cream
1 cup grated Parmesan
    cheese

Quick vegetarian lasagna

* Preheat the oven to 425°F.

* Heat the oil in a frying pan. Add the onion and sauté for 5 minutes, or until starting to soften. Add the chiles and garlic and sauté for 1 minute. Add the mushrooms and sauté for 2 minutes, then add the roasted red peppers and spinach and toss together. Add the tomatoes and tomato paste, and season with salt and pepper. Simmer for 2 to 3 minutes, then remove from the heat and add the basil.

* Soak the lasagna noodles in hot water for 5 minutes, then drain.

* To make the sauce, melt the butter in a saucepan. Add the flour and whisk together to make a smooth roux. Blend in the milk and crème fraîche. Season with salt and pepper and add half the Parmesan.

* Put a third of the vegetables in an ovenproof dish. Pour in a third of the sauce, then top with 2 of the lasagna noodles. Spoon in half of the remaining vegetables and half of the remaining sauce. Put the remaining 2 lasagna noodles on top and spoon on the remaining vegetables and sauce. Sprinkle with the remaining Parmesan.

* Bake for 25 to 30 minutes, until golden and bubbling.

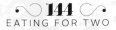

Roasted vegetables make a simple but delicious sauce for pasta. For a tasty alternative, you could also mix the vegetables with couscous.

• • •

MAKES 3 PORTIONS

1 small eggplant, coarsely chopped
1 medium zucchini, chopped
4 large plum tomatoes, each cut into 6 wedges
1 red onion, cut into 12 wedges
1 yellow or red bell pepper, seeded and cut into ¾-inch pieces
2 cloves garlic
1½ tablespoons fresh thyme leaves
1½ tablespoons olive oil
Salt and pepper
8 ounces fusilli pasta
1½ tablespoons good-quality balsamic vinegar
5 tablespoons grated Parmesan cheese
3 tablespoons chopped fresh basil

Pasta with roasted vegetables, balsamic vinegar, and basil

✳ **RICH IN FOLIC ACID** ✳

✳ Preheat the oven to 400°F.

✳ Place all the vegetables in a roasting pan together with the garlic cloves. Sprinkle with the thyme and olive oil and season with salt and pepper. Place in the oven for 30 minutes, turning halfway through. While the vegetables are roasting, cook the pasta following the package instructions.

✳ Stir the balsamic vinegar into the vegetables and then toss with the drained pasta. Finally, stir in the Parmesan and fresh basil.

½ large butternut squash,
    peeled, seeded, and
    cut into ½-inch cubes
3 tablespoons olive oil
1 large red onion, root end
    left intact, cut lengthwise
    into 12 wedges
2 heaping tablespoons
    pumpkin seeds
2 tablespoons canola oil
1 tablespoon rice vinegar
½ teaspoon soy sauce
1 teaspoon sugar
1 teaspoon mirin (or use
    ¼ teaspoon extra sugar)
4 cups (loosely packed)
    mizuna or arugula leaves

Roasted
squash salad with
pumpkin seeds

✳ Preheat the oven to 400°F.

✳ Put the squash in a bowl, drizzle with 2 tablespoons of the olive oil, and toss to coat the squash cubes. Spread out on a large baking sheet and roast for 40 to 45 minutes, turning every 10 minutes, until soft and browned at the edges.

✳ While the squash is cooking, toss the onion with the remaining 1 tablespoon oil and put on a small baking sheet. Roast for 10 to 15 minutes, until soft. Toast the pumpkin seeds in a dry frying pan for 5 minutes. Transfer to a plate to cool slightly.

✳ Whisk the canola oil, vinegar, soy sauce, sugar, and mirin, if using, in a small bowl. Put the mizuna or arugula leaves in a large bowl and add the squash and onion. Pour on the dressing and gently toss. Scatter with the pumpkin seeds and serve immediately.

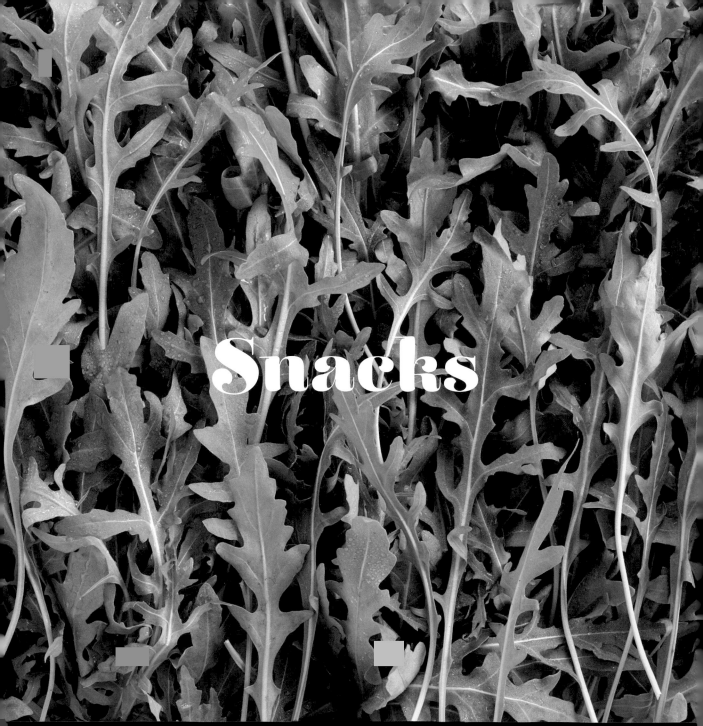

Snacks

Scant 1 cup boiling water
1 or 2 slices lemon
2 slices peeled fresh ginger
4 sprigs fresh mint
½ to 1 teaspoon honey

Infused ginger
and lemon tea

✳ Measure the boiling water into a teapot. Add the lemon, ginger, and mint. Let infuse for 5 minutes, then pour through a small strainer into a cup. Stir in the honey to taste.

✳ If you like a stronger flavor, add the lemon and ginger to the cup.

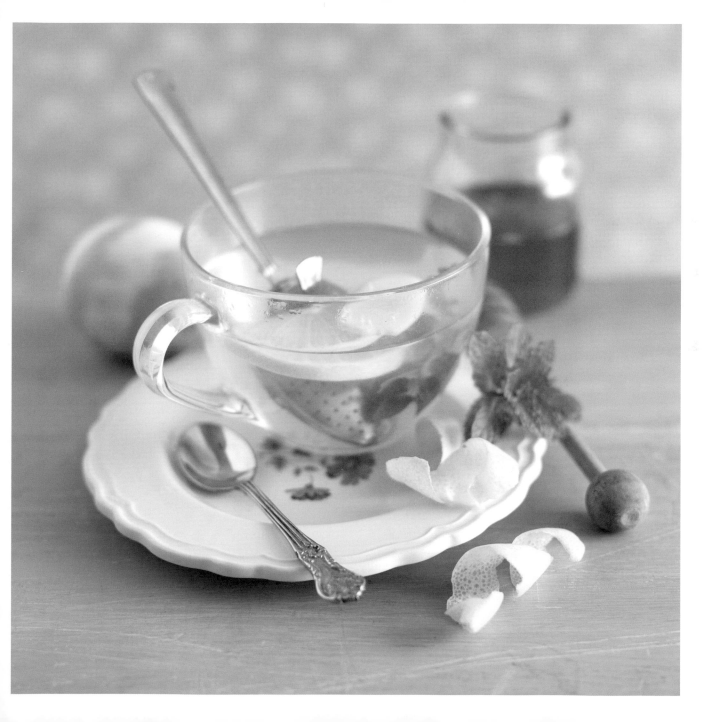

½ large ripe mango, diced
½ banana, sliced
⅓ cup mango or
　　tropical-fruit yogurt
2 tablespoons apple juice
Honey (optional)

Mango and banana smoothie

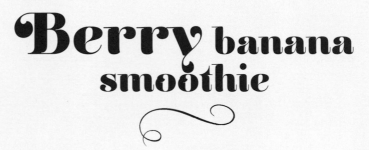

✷ Blend the mango and banana until smooth. Add the yogurt and juice and blend until just combined. Stir in honey to taste if the smoothie needs extra sweetness.

MAKES 1 SMOOTHIE

¾ cup raspberries
½ banana, sliced
½ cup strawberry yogurt
　　drink or strawberry yogurt
Honey (optional)

Berry banana smoothie

✷ Blend the raspberries and banana until smooth. Add the yogurt and blend until just combined. Stir in honey to taste if the smoothie needs extra sweetness.

✷ Prepare ahead: You can put fruit in bags (already portioned) and freeze. Take out of the freezer and let stand for about 5 minutes before blending.

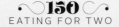

1 cup all-purpose flour
¾ cup plus 1 tablespoon
　 whole wheat flour
1 teaspoon ground ginger
1 teaspoon ground
　 cinnamon
2 teaspoons baking powder
¾ teaspoon baking soda
Generous pinch of salt
½ cup raisins
2¼ cups grated carrots
¾ cup plain whole milk
　 yogurt
1 egg
⅓ cup canola oil
1 teaspoon vanilla extract
¾ cup (firmly packed) light
　 brown sugar
2 tablespoons maple syrup
1 tablespoon sunflower
　 seeds

Carrot and raisin muffins

✳ Preheat the oven to 375°F. Line a muffin pan with paper cases.

✳ Put the flours, ginger, cinnamon, baking powder, baking soda, and salt in a bowl and mix together. Stir in the raisins, followed by the carrots.

✳ Whisk together the yogurt, egg, oil, vanilla extract, sugar, and syrup. Stir into the carrot mixture until just combined. Divide among the muffin cups and sprinkle the sunflower seeds on top.

✳ Bake for 20 to 22 minutes, until risen and firm to the touch. Let cool in the pan for 10 minutes, then transfer to a wire rack to cool completely.

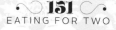

Pumpkin seeds are a good source of essential fatty acids, iron, and zinc, and sunflower seeds are rich in vitamins E and B. This makes a tasty and nutritious snack.

• • •

MAKES ABOUT 1 CUP

1 tablespoon canola oil
½ cup pumpkin seeds
½ cup sunflower seeds
1 tablespoon honey
1 tablespoon soy sauce

Honey and SOY toasted seeds

✱ Heat the canola oil in a nonstick frying pan, then add the pumpkin and sunflower seeds and cook, stirring continuously, for about 2 minutes, or until the seeds are lightly browned. Remove from the heat, stir in the honey and soy sauce, and return to the heat for 1 minute. Spread the seeds out on a nonstick baking sheet and let cool. When cool, store in an airtight container.

MAKES ABOUT 1 CUP

Small pat of butter
Scant 1 cup pecan halves
3 tablespoons pumpkin seeds
2 teaspoons turbinado sugar

Glazed pecans and pumpkin seeds

✱ Melt the butter in a small frying pan. Add the pecan halves and pumpkin seeds and lightly toast in the pan. Add the sugar and toss together over the heat for 1 minute. Let cool.

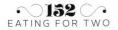

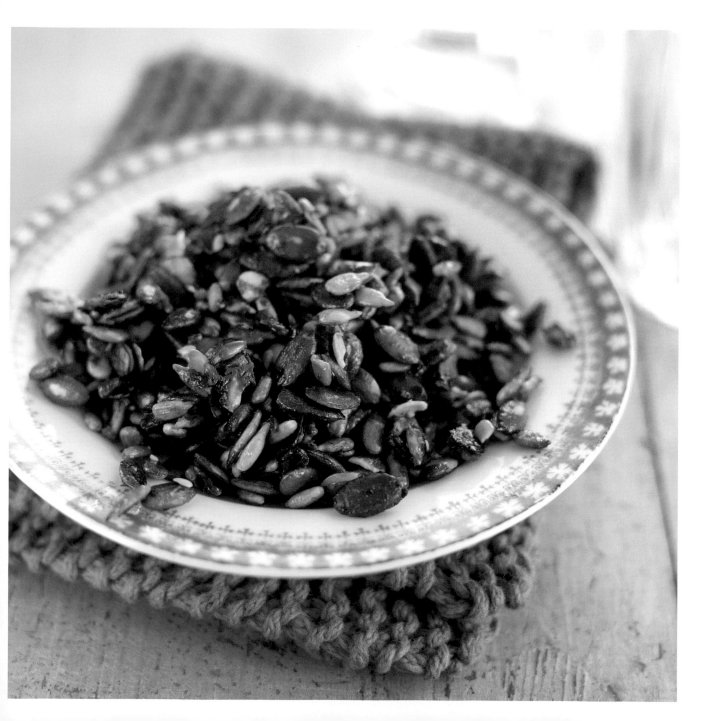

1 tablespoon olive oil

2 medium onions, thinly
   sliced

Leaves from 2 sprigs of fresh
   thyme

1½ teaspoons balsamic
   vinegar

1 teaspoon honey

Salt and pepper

4 flour tortillas

1⅓ cups (loosely packed)
   shredded cooked chicken

1 cup grated Cheddar or
   Monterey Jack cheese

Chicken quesadillas with caramelized onion

✳ Heat the oil in a frying pan. Add the onions and thyme and cook, stirring frequently, for 20 to 25 minutes over medium-low heat, until the onions are soft and golden. Add the vinegar and honey and cook for 1 minute, or until the vinegar has evaporated. Season to taste with salt and pepper and set aside to cool slightly. Divide the onion mixture between 2 of the tortillas and spread out. Top with the chicken and cheese and sandwich with the remaining 2 tortillas.

✳ Preheat a large nonstick frying pan over medium heat. Slide in one assembled quesadilla, cheese side down, and cook for 1 to 2 minutes. Flip onto the other side and heat through for 1 more minute. Transfer to a plate and let stand for 3 to 5 minutes before cutting, to stop the cheese from oozing out. Repeat with the remaining assembled quesadillas.

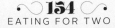

1 tablespoon olive oil
1⅓ cups thinly sliced
   cremini mushrooms
Leaves from 1 sprig of fresh
   thyme
1 scallion, thinly sliced
½ clove garlic, crushed
Salt and pepper
2 flour tortillas
½ cup grated Gruyère cheese

Mushroom and Gruyère quesadilla

✷ Heat the oil in a frying pan. Add the mushrooms and thyme leaves and sauté for 6 to 8 minutes, until the mushrooms are golden.

✷ Add the scallion and garlic and sauté for 1 to 2 minutes more, until the scallion softens. Remove from the heat. Season to taste with salt and pepper and let cool slightly. Spread over one of the tortillas, scatter the Gruyère on top, and sandwich with the remaining tortilla.

✷ Preheat a large nonstick frying pan over medium heat. Slide in the assembled quesadilla, cheese side down, and cook for 1 to 2 minutes. Flip onto the other side and heat through for 1 more minute. Transfer to a plate and let stand for 3 to 5 minutes before cutting, to stop the cheese from oozing out.

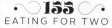

1 teaspoon whole-grain
   mustard
½ teaspoon honey
2 flour tortillas
2 or 3 thin slices smoked
   ham (about 1 ounce)
½ cup grated sharp Cheddar
   cheese

Ham and honey mustard quesadilla

✶ Mix the mustard and honey together and spread over one of the tortillas. Lay the ham on top and sprinkle with the Cheddar. Sandwich with the second tortilla.

✶ Preheat a large nonstick frying pan over medium heat. Slide in the assembled quesadilla, cheese side down, and cook for 1 to 2 minutes. Flip onto the other side and heat through for 1 minute more. Remove from the pan and let stand on a plate for 3 to 5 minutes before cutting, to stop the cheese from oozing out.

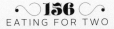

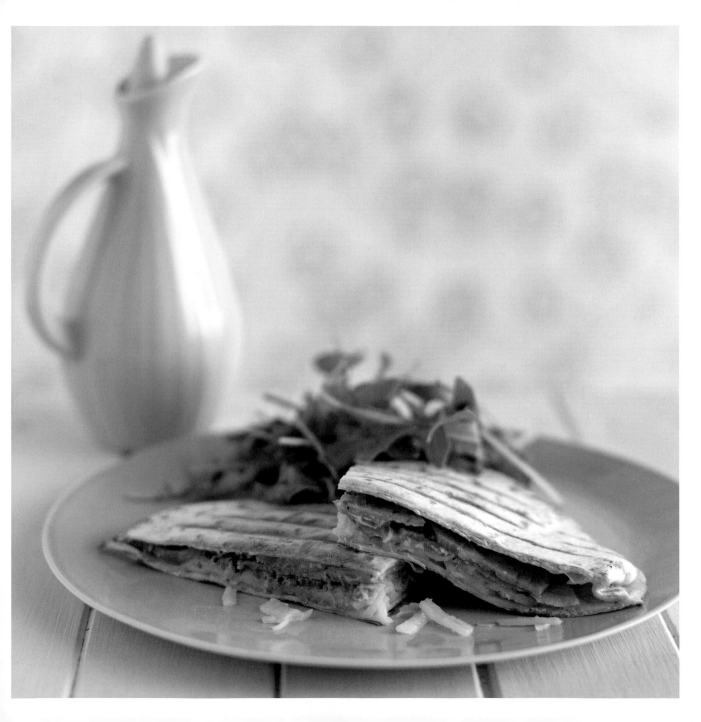

2 flour tortillas
2 tablespoons light
   mayonnaise
4 thin slices of pastrami
1 dill pickle, thinly sliced
1 tomato, seeded and sliced
Handful of shredded lettuce
Salt and pepper

Pastrami, dill pickle, and tomato wrap

✳ Warm the tortillas in the microwave for 20 seconds and place on a cutting board. Spread 1 tablespoon of the mayonnaise along one side of each tortilla. Top each tortilla with 2 slices pastrami, half the sliced dill pickle, half the sliced tomato, and half the lettuce. Season with salt and pepper, then roll up. Slice each wrap in half diagonally.

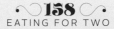

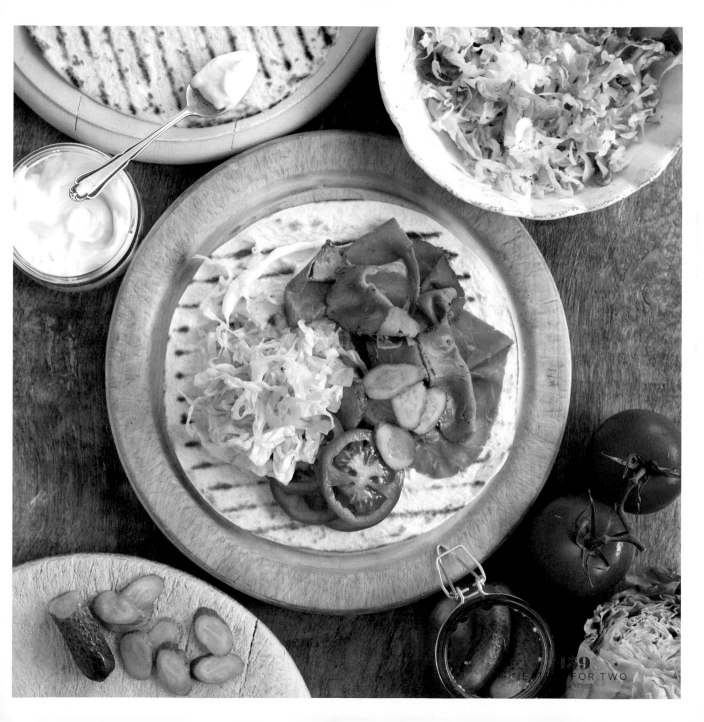

2 flour tortillas
2 tablespoons light
    mayonnaise
¼ cup mango chutney
½ cooked chicken breast,
    sliced
Handful of arugula
3 tablespoons diced fresh
    mango
Salt and pepper

Mango, chicken, and arugula wrap

✻ Warm the tortillas in the microwave for 20 seconds.
Spread 1 tablespoon of the mayonnaise onto each tortilla.
Spread 2 tablespoons of the mango chutney on top of the
mayonnaise. Top each tortilla with half of the sliced
chicken, arugula, and mango. Season with salt and pepper
and roll up. Slice in half diagonally.

MAKES ABOUT 1½ CUPS

One 15-ounce can
    chickpeas, drained and
    rinsed
½ cup drained bottled
    roasted red peppers,
    chopped
1 clove garlic, crushed
3 tablespoons olive oil
2 tablespoons Greek yogurt
Juice of half a lemon
Pinch of sugar
Salt and pepper
Pita bread

Red pepper hummus

✻ Put the chickpeas, red peppers, and garlic in a food
processor. Whiz until finely chopped. While the processor
is running, drizzle in the oil. Add the yogurt, lemon juice,
and sugar. Season well with salt and pepper. Whiz again
until smooth. Serve with warm pita bread.

2 English muffins
Butter
¼ cup tomato paste
1 tablespoon olive oil
1 small red onion, sliced
1 cup thinly sliced button
    mushrooms
⅓ cup drained bottled
    roasted red peppers,
    coarsely chopped
1 tomato, thinly sliced
½ cup grated Cheddar
    cheese
Salt and pepper

English muffin pizzas

✳ Split the muffins in half. Toast in a toaster until golden. Spread with a little butter and then spread 1 tablespoon of the tomato paste over each muffin half. Place on a baking sheet and preheat the broiler.

✳ Heat the oil in a saucepan. Add the onion and sauté for 3 minutes. Add the mushrooms and sauté for another 2 to 3 minutes, then remove from the heat. Divide the mixture among the muffins. Top with the peppers and sliced tomato, then sprinkle with the Cheddar. Season with salt and pepper. Place under the broiler for 4 to 5 minutes, until the cheese is melted and lightly golden on top.

3 ounces green beans, cut into thirds

Pat of butter

Scant ½ cup pecan halves

3 tablespoons superfine sugar

1 small head red leaf lettuce, leaves roughly torn

1 cup (loosely packed) arugula leaves

2 large tomatoes, sliced

2 tablespoons drained canned corn

3 tablespoons olive oil

2 teaspoons good-quality aged balsamic vinegar

2 teaspoons granulated sugar

½ teaspoon Dijon mustard

1½ tablespoons soy sauce

Salad of green beans, pecans, and tomatoes with soy and balsamic dressing

✳ Cook the green beans in boiling salted water for 3 minutes. Drain and refresh in cold water.

✳ Melt the butter in a frying pan. Add the pecans and sprinkle with the superfine sugar. Toss together over the heat until the sugar has melted and coated the pecans. Let cool.

✳ Arrange the lettuce and arugula on a plate. Top with the tomatoes and sprinkle with the corn, pecan halves, and beans.

✳ To make the dressing, mix together the olive oil, vinegar, granulated sugar, mustard, and soy sauce. Pour over the salad.

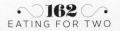

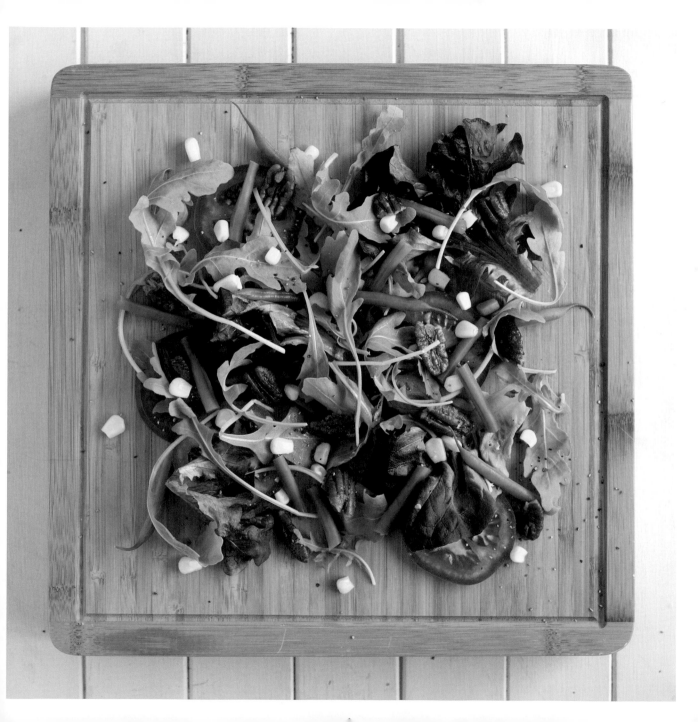

5: And Then There Were Two

Nutrition after your baby arrives

Congratulations! After (approximately) nine months, you've finally met your lovely baby. Your good nutrition and care have helped your baby develop and grow, but for (hopefully) most of you, the job is not over yet. If you're breast-feeding, you will continue to be your baby's only or main source of nutrition for up to six months—it's a huge responsibility. Your baby's weight gain will continue to zoom upward: He will more than double his birth weight in these first six months of life, often nourished only by your breast milk. This means continuing to eat well, both for your baby and for yourself. And one more job: Whether you're breast-feeding or not, shedding those excess pregnancy pounds will pay health dividends for years to come.

Nutrition priorities during breast-feeding

If you're breast-feeding, your body's requirements will increase by the calories and other nutrients needed to produce breast milk. Amazingly, your body will be producing an average of 3½ cups of milk per day if you are exclusively breast-feeding, which requires an extra 675 calories a day. However, you don't need to get all these extra calories from your diet—many will come from the fat stores your body put away during pregnancy for just this purpose, meaning breast-feeding will give a great boost to shedding those pregnancy pounds.

It's not just calories that are needed—your body's requirement for a raft of different nutrients increases. Continue to follow the balanced diet outlined in chapter 1 and you will meet most of these needs. However, there are a few nutrients you might need to think about in particular:

Calcium

It's hardly surprising that the requirement for calcium increases when breast-feeding. Aim for 4 or 5 servings of dairy foods or other calcium-rich foods each day. See page 18 for more on calcium.

Vitamin D

Vitamin D is another nutrient that can fall short when breast-feeding. It's recommended that you continue the 10 mcg per day vitamin D supplement you've been taking during pregnancy.

Omega-3s

Omega-3 fats continue to be important—they provide a component of your baby's brain, eyes, and nerves, which continue to grow and develop after birth. Continue to eat oil-rich fish, though not more than two portions per week. Please note that the FDA and EPA tell nursing mothers to avoid shark, swordfish, king mackerel, and tilefish.

Fluid

Another thing you'll need more of is fluid. From just a few tablespoons of breast milk in the early days of breast-feeding, you may go on to produce up to 3½ cups per day. While you're breast-feeding, your fluid requirement skyrockets to about 12 glasses per day. You can meet this by having a drink at each meal or snack, and when breast-feeding. Keep a bottle of water handy wherever you tend to breast-feed. You'll be surprised how thirsty you get.

What if I'm a vegetarian or vegan and breast-feeding?

Just as during pregnancy, a vegetarian or vegan diet can be perfectly healthy for breast-feeding, provided it is well planned. Again, the nutrients at risk include vitamin B_{12}, vitamin D, and omega-3 oils. If you're a vegan, you'll also need to think about vitamin B_2 and calcium, as well as eating a variety of plant-based proteins each day. Refer back to the section on being pregnant and vegetarian (see page 30), as well as Pregnancy Supernutrients (see page 16), for more on all these nutrients. Also remember that it's important to continue your vitamin D supplement.

Weight loss

After having a baby, you'll continue to look pregnant for a while. You'll have lost the weight of your baby, the amniotic fluid, and the placenta, but it takes time for your uterus to contract and shrink. You will still have larger breasts and the extra pounds gained to support breast-feeding. However, it's beneficial to try to return to your normal healthy weight range, especially if you want to try to conceive again.

It's important to remember that your body will still be recovering from the birth, and this may take a while. Wait for at least a month after the birth before attempting to lose any weight. Then reread the guidelines in chapter 1 on a balanced diet, and watch out for high-fat and high-sugar foods that contain plenty of calories but few nutrients. A little gentle exercise will also help—walking while pushing your baby in his stroller, for example.

Losing weight while breast-feeding

If you are breast-feeding, you'll need to take in enough calories and other nutrients to support this. You'll need a diet that provides for your needs as well; otherwise, you risk depriving your own body in order to provide the nutrients for your baby. If you are breast-feeding, you'll burn many more calories than if you weren't, giving a boost to any weight-loss efforts.

As always, eat a healthy, low-fat, low-sugar diet that follows the recommendations in chapter 1. You'll also need another few servings of dairy foods, as outlined on page 164. It is safe to lose weight while breast-feeding, but you should do so slowly: Studies have shown that gradual weight loss of up to a pound a week does not interfere with milk production or your baby's weight gain. If you find you are losing weight faster than this, try to eat a little more, maybe by adding an extra snack.

To keep hunger pangs at bay while breast-feeding, eat regular healthy snacks. Follow the guidelines on controlling your appetite on page 70.

Losing weight if not breast-feeding

Because you don't have the additional demands of breast-feeding on your body, you can follow a normal weight-loss plan once your body has recovered from the birth. In practice this is similar to if you're breast-feeding, because you continue to follow recommendations for eating from the food groups (though only 2 or 3 servings of dairy foods or nondairy equivalents are required each day). It's always sensible to aim for weight loss at a modest speed: About 1 to 2 pounds a week is a healthy rate. Depriving yourself of too many calories would risk leaving you without enough energy to look after yourself and your new baby.

Thinking about allergies

Official advice regarding allergies has changed in the last few years. There's no clear evidence that avoiding peanuts while breast-feeding alters your baby's chance of developing allergies. Therefore it's no longer recommended that nuts or other allergens should be avoided, unless either the mother or the baby has an allergy. Occasionally there is a situation in which a mother needs to avoid allergenic foods, such as dairy products, because her baby has an allergy, but you should not do this unless it's recommended by a dietitian, a pediatrician, or another health care provider.

Alcohol and caffeine

While you wouldn't choose to feed alcohol or caffeine to your new baby, it's important to remember that they both pass in small amounts from your body into your breast milk. Thus they still need to be limited—yes, even after the birth!

Alcohol

While many women choose not to drink alcohol while breast-feeding, research suggests that drinking small amounts (no more than one drink per day) is unlikely to harm your baby. Each drink will take up to two hours to clear from your system, so try to time your drink to allow a few hours before breast-feeding. Another option is to express milk for your baby before drinking, if you expect to have a drink or two.

Caffeine

As adults we drink caffeine to keep us awake. While it's the last thing we want to do to our babies, caffeine passing through your breast milk can have this effect. To avoid this, it's recommended that you drink caffeinated drinks such as tea, coffee, and cola only occasionally, rather than every day, while your baby is breast-feeding. Decaffeinated coffee and tea as well as fruit teas are fine to consume as you wish.

Can certain foods upset my baby if I'm breast-feeding?

Spicy foods; "gassy" vegetables such as cabbage, beans, onions, and brussels sprouts; and citrus fruits are notorious for causing problems for breast-feeding babies. Can this really be possible? Well, it's known that food molecules (and food flavors) do pass from a mother's diet to the baby through breast milk. That said, most women eat a varied diet, including so-called problem foods, and their babies experience no adverse effects, so there's usually no need to avoid anything.

However, if you find there are certain foods that seem to cause your baby problems, and they are easily replaced by other foods from the same food group, feel free to skip them. If you feel that foods that make up a major part of your diet may be causing problems, speak to your pediatrician.

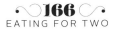

Desserts

This is one of my favorite crumbles—it is so simple to make but utterly delicious. I like to serve it hot with vanilla ice cream.

•••

MAKES 4 PORTIONS

Scant 1½ cups all-purpose flour

5 tablespoons butter, cut into cubes

¼ cup quick-cooking oats

2 tablespoons chopped pecans

¼ cup turbinado sugar

2 cups fresh blackberries

2 cups fresh raspberries

3 tablespoons granulated sugar

Raspberry and blackberry crumble

∗ Preheat the oven to 400°F.

∗ To make the topping, combine the flour and butter in a bowl. Rub together using your fingers until the mixture looks like bread crumbs. Work in the oats, pecans, and turbinado sugar.

∗ Put the blackberries and raspberries in a small, shallow baking dish. Sprinkle with the granulated sugar, then the topping. Bake for 30 to 35 minutes, until bubbling and lightly golden on top.

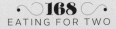

Chocolate and prunes combine to make these delectable brownies. Some people crave chocolate when they are pregnant. I know I did! Maybe it's because when you eat chocolate, it causes the brain to release chemicals that make you feel good.

• • •

Chocolate and prune
brownies

MAKES 12 BROWNIES
SUITABLE FOR FREEZING

10 ounces good-quality bittersweet chocolate, chopped
2 sticks plus 1 tablespoon butter, cut into cubes
6 eggs
1¼ cups superfine sugar
3 tablespoons unsweetened cocoa powder
5 tablespoons self-rising flour
½ cup finely chopped prunes

✴ Preheat the oven to 350°F.

✴ Line an 8-inch square cake pan with parchment paper and grease well.

✴ Put the chocolate and butter into a heatproof bowl. Melt over a pan of simmering water, stirring until smooth. Let cool slightly.

✴ Beat the eggs and sugar in a bowl. Whisk in the melted chocolate and butter. Sift in the cocoa powder and flour, mix well, then stir in the prunes. Pour into the pan and level the top. Bake for 45 minutes, or until well risen around the edges with a slight wobble in the middle. Let cool in the pan for 1 hour before slicing.

Tip
Why not enjoy these brownies with some fresh berries for additional fiber and vitamins?

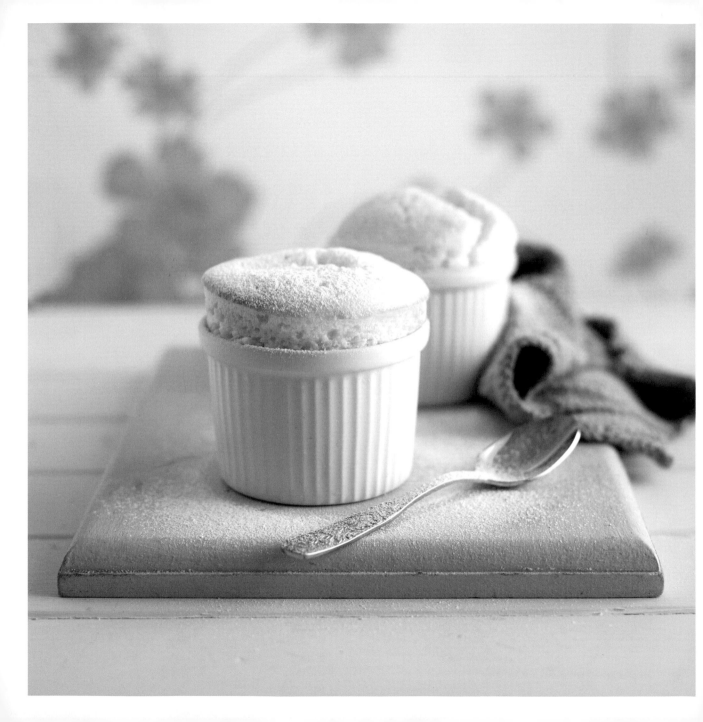

This is heavenly and
oh-so-simple to prepare . . .
treat yourself!

• • •

MAKES 6 PORTIONS

½ cup butter, softened
½ cup superfine sugar
4 eggs, separated
5 tablespoons all-purpose
   flour
Finely grated zest and juice
   of 2 large lemons
1¼ cups milk

Lemon soufflé pudding

✴ Preheat the oven to 350°F. Grease a 1½-quart ovenproof
dish or six 1-cup ramekins.

✴ Whisk the butter and sugar in a bowl until light and fluffy.
Add the egg yolks, flour, and lemon zest and juice, and
whisk again. Slowly add the milk to make a thick batter.
The mixture will look curdled at this point.

✴ Whisk the egg whites until stiff, then fold into the lemon
mixture. Pour into the prepared dish or ramekins. Bake for
30 minutes, or until lightly golden and well risen on top.

1¼ cups sliced strawberries
¾ cup blueberries
1¼ cups Greek-style yogurt
¼ cup turbinado sugar
¾ cup crushed amaretti
   cookies

Brûlée-style strawberry dessert

★ RICH IN VITAMIN C ★

★ Put the strawberries and blueberries in the bottom of four 6-ounce glass ramekins or larger wineglasses. Spoon the yogurt on top. Sprinkle with the turbinado sugar and top with the crushed amaretti. Refrigerate for 1 hour.

Tip

Berries are a delicious source of vitamin C. As well as being vital in its own right, vitamin C increases the absorption of iron in plant foods, such as green leafy vegetables, lentils, nuts, and seeds, eaten at the same time, as well as the iron in eggs.

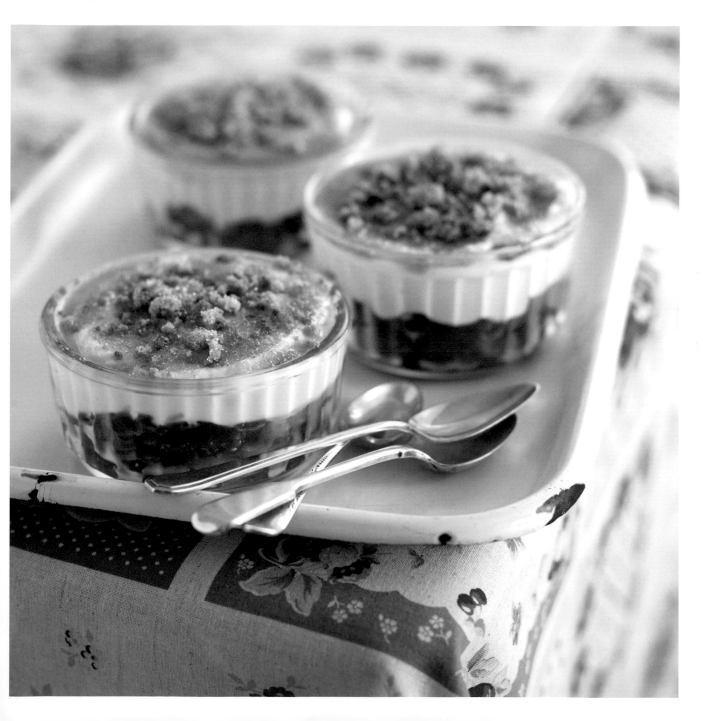

Try this easy version of
the classic dessert.

• • •

MAKES 4 TO 6 PORTIONS

2 tablespoons decaffeinated
coffee granules
Scant 1 cup boiling water
16 ladyfingers
½ cup mascarpone
2 tablespoons confectioners'
sugar
1¼ cups good-quality ready-
to-eat vanilla pudding
1 teaspoon vanilla extract
Unsweetened cocoa powder

Tiramisù

✳ Dissolve the coffee granules in the boiling water and pour
into a shallow dish. Dip the ladyfingers into the coffee and
arrange 8 ladyfingers in the base of a small dish or divide
among four to six dessert dishes. Mix the mascarpone, confectioners' sugar, and vanilla pudding together, then whisk
until smooth. Whisk in the vanilla extract. Spread half the
mixture over the ladyfingers. Sprinkle with cocoa powder,
then put another layer of ladyfingers on top and spread
with the remaining mascarpone mixture. Sprinkle with
cocoa powder. Refrigerate for 2 hours, or overnight if
possible.

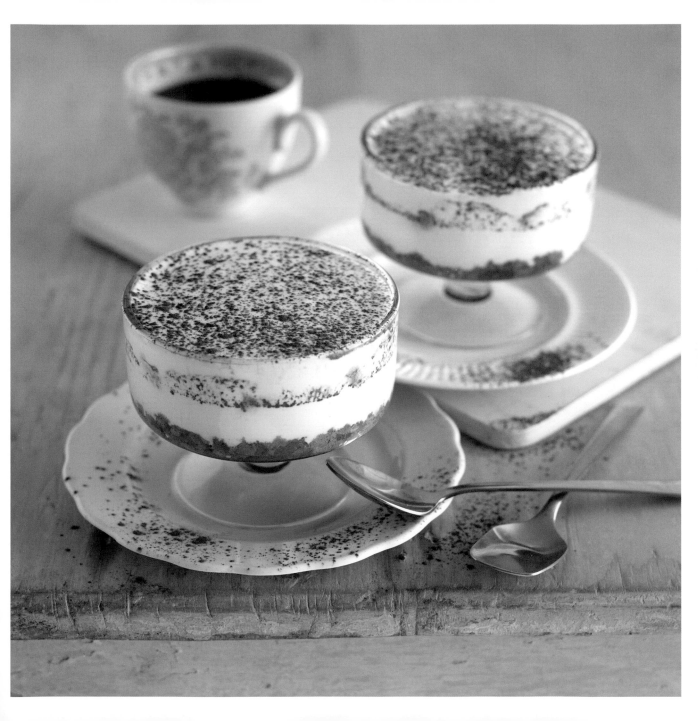

Having a bowl of this deliciously refreshing dessert is a perfect way to cool down on a hot day.

• • •

MAKES 6 PORTIONS

1¼ cups sugar
2½ cups water
4 large lemons
2 cups raspberries,
  to serve

Lemon granita

✶ Put the sugar and water in a saucepan. Stir over low heat until dissolved. Let cool. Grate the zest from one of the lemons and add to the syrup. Juice all of the lemons and add to the syrup. Stir and pour into a shallow plastic container. Place in the freezer until frozen, stirring from time to time. Spoon into glasses and serve with the raspberries.

✶ The granita should have a rough, crystal-like consistency. It should not be smooth like a sorbet.

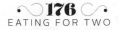

8 tablespoons (1 stick)
   butter, softened
⅔ cup (tightly packed) light
   brown sugar
1 egg, beaten
Scant 1 cup all-purpose flour
1⅔ cups quick-cooking oats
¾ cup golden raisins
½ teaspoon baking powder
½ teaspoon pumpkin pie
   spice
1 teaspoon vanilla extract

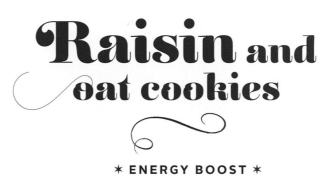

Raisin and oat cookies

✶ ENERGY BOOST ✶

✶ Preheat the oven to 350°F. Grease 2 baking sheets.

✶ Whisk the butter and sugar together. Add the egg and whisk again. Add the remaining ingredients and mix until combined.

✶ Shape into 18 little cookies. Arrange on the baking sheets and press down to flatten. Bake for 18 minutes.

Tip

Oats are a great addition to anyone's diet. As well as providing valuable fiber, they release their energy slowly to keep you going longer.

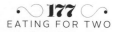

This is one of my favorite desserts. It is good served warm or cold, and the fruit compote has a wonderful flavor due to the rosewater. The pomegranates add a crunchy texture that complements the berries beautifully.

• • •

MAKES 4 PORTIONS

1 large ripe peach
2 large red plums
1½ tablespoons butter
2 tablespoons sugar
1 tablespoon rosewater or orange flower water (can also use plain water)
⅔ cup raspberries
Scant ½ cup red currants
⅔ cup blackberries
Seeds of 1 pomegranate

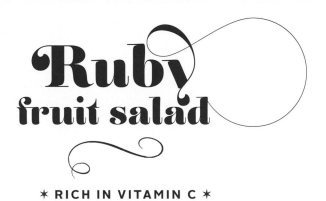

Ruby fruit salad

✳ RICH IN VITAMIN C ✳

✳ Halve the peach and plums, remove the pits, and cut each half into four pieces. Melt the butter in a large frying pan and place the plum and peach slices in the butter.

✳ Cook for 2 to 3 minutes before flipping over and sprinkling with the sugar. Cook for 2 to 3 minutes more and then pour in the rosewater. Gently stir in the remaining fruits and heat through for approximately 1 minute. Divide among four dessert dishes.

Superfood

Berries are rich in vitamin C, which is needed for growth and also helps iron absorption. Vitamin C is water soluble and cannot be stored in the body, so foods containing vitamin C should be eaten every day.

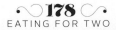

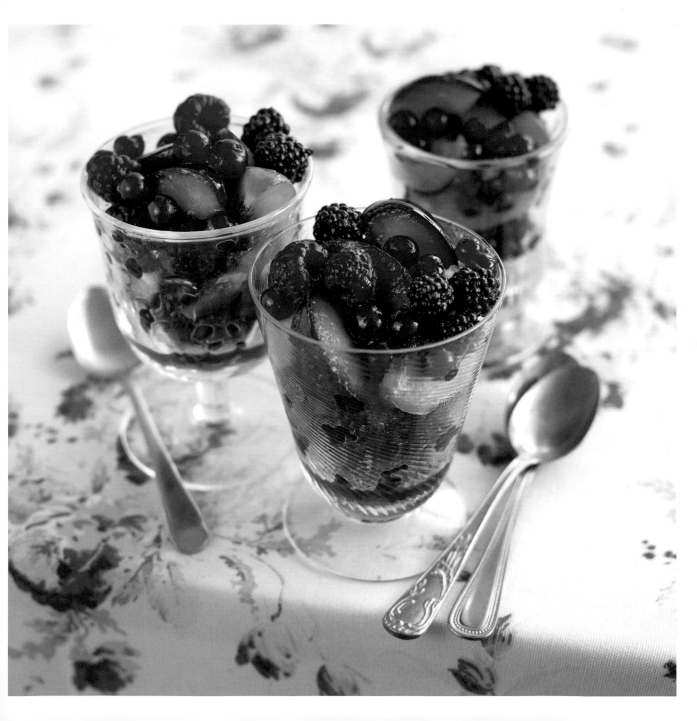

Desserts are usually thought of as the bad guys of the nutrition world. However, by choosing wisely, such as with this delicious fruit compote, your dessert bowl can be a source of fiber and rich in vitamins. Add some low-fat yogurt and you'll also gain bone-building calcium.

• • •

MAKES 2 PORTIONS

2 ripe peaches
2 large ripe plums
Pat of butter
⅓ cup blueberries
1½ to 2 tablespoons sugar

Peach and plum compote

✳ Slice the peaches and plums in half and remove the pits. Slice the peaches into 8 wedges and the plums into quarters.

✳ Heat the butter in a saucepan. Add the fruit and lightly toss in the butter. Sprinkle with the sugar and continue to stir over the heat for another minute. Spoon into serving bowls.

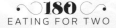

It's easy to make your own fruit gelatin using fruit juice and powdered gelatin.

• • •

MAKES 4 PORTIONS

One ¼-ounce envelope unflavored gelatin

1¼ cups white grape juice

¾ cup cranberry juice cocktail

⅓ cup sugar

⅔ cup raspberries

½ cup quartered strawberries

Fruity Cranberry Gelatin

✳ Put 2 tablespoons water in a small bowl and sprinkle with the gelatin. Let stand for 10 minutes.

✳ Combine the grape and cranberry juices with the sugar in a saucepan and heat gently, stirring occasionally, until hot and the sugar has dissolved. Remove the saucepan from the heat, add the gelatin, and stir until the gelatin has dissolved. Let cool.

✳ Divide the fruit among four glasses. Pour the juice mixture over the fruit, put in the refrigerator, and let set for about 6 hours or, preferably, overnight.

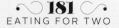

This is a wonderful cake to make when you have friends over, or for a special occasion such as a bridal or baby shower.

•••

3 eggs
1⅓ cups self-rising flour
12 tablespoons (1½ sticks) butter, softened
¾ cup plus 2 tablespoons superfine sugar
1 teaspoon baking powder
2 tablespoons strong brewed coffee

Frosting
6½ tablespoons salted butter, softened
2 cups confectioners' sugar
1 tablespoon strong brewed coffee
Heaping ⅓ cup walnut halves, coarsely chopped

Coffee and walnut cake

✳ Preheat the oven to 350°F. Line and grease an 8-inch round cake pan.

✳ Put the eggs, flour, butter, sugar, baking powder, and coffee into a bowl and beat together using a handheld electric mixer until blended. Spoon into the pan and level the top. Bake in the oven for 35 to 40 minutes, until well risen and shrinking away from the sides of the pan. Transfer to a wire rack and let cool in the pan.

✳ To make the frosting, beat the butter and confectioners' sugar together using a handheld electric mixer until light and fluffy. Beat in the coffee. Frost the top of the cake and sprinkle with the walnuts.

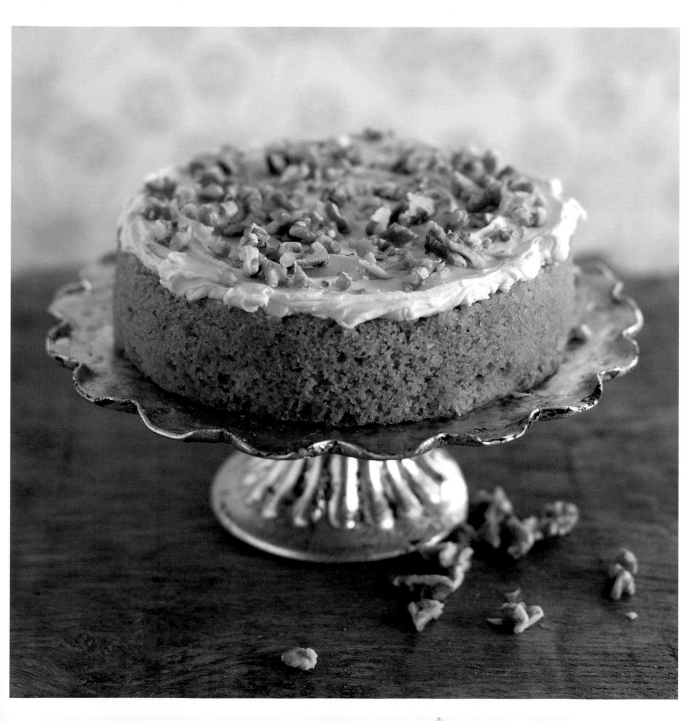

9 double graham crackers, crushed (18 squares, to make 1½ cups)

5 tablespoons butter, melted

8 ounces cream cheese, at room temperature

Scant 1 cup heavy cream

½ cup lemon curd (can be found in the jams and jellies aisle of your market)

Juice and zest of half a small lemon

Fresh berries (optional)

Lemon cheesecake

✻ You will need an 8-inch springform pan. Grease the base and line with parchment paper.

✻ Mix the graham cracker crumbs and butter together. Press into the base of the pan and refrigerate for 30 minutes.

✻ Put the cream cheese and heavy cream into a bowl and beat with a handheld electric mixer until lightly whipped. Add the lemon curd and the lemon juice and zest. Mix until smooth and thickened. Spoon into the pan and level the top. Refrigerate for 2 hours, or until set.

✻ Serve with fresh berries if you like.

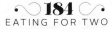

Index

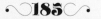

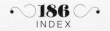

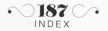

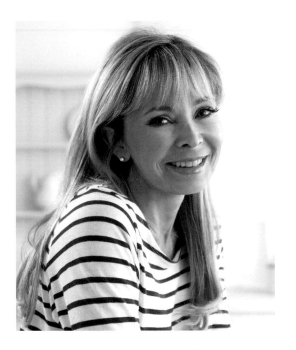

Annabel Karmel is a mother of three and bestselling author of twenty-five books on feeding babies and children (as well as teaching children how to cook). Her books have sold more than 4 million copies worldwide. She is well known for providing advice and guidance for millions of parents all over the world on what to feed their children, as well as getting families to eat a healthier diet without spending hours in the kitchen. Annabel travels frequently to the United States and has appeared on many TV shows, including *The View, Live with Regis and Kelly,* and the *Today* show.

In 2006, Annabel was awarded an MBE (Member of the British Empire) by Queen Elizabeth for her services to nutrition for children, and in 2010, she won the media category of the First Women Awards, which recognize women at the top of their professions who are leading the way for the next generation. Her website, www.annabelkarmel.com, is the number one site for delicious recipes for babies, children, and adults, as well as information on all aspects of nutrition. She also has a successful iPhone app, "Annabel Karmel's Essential Guide to Feeding Your Baby & Toddler," with more than 120 recipes and videos, and a popular children's cooking TV show, *Annabel's Kitchen,* which is loved by moms and kids, as a well as a range of healthy Disney snacks for toddlers.

www.annabelkarmel.com

Acknowledgments

I would like to thank the following for their help and work on this book: Dave King, for his wonderful photography; Smith & Gilmour, for their inspired design; Kate Blinman, for food, and Jo Harris, for props; Fiona Hinton, for her superb knowledge and advice; Lucinda Kaicik; Jonathan Lloyd; Stephen Margolis; Mary Jones; Evelyn Etkind; and Alice Fotheringham. Also Erica Auger, for kindly allowing her "bump" to be featured! And to the Ebury team: Carey Smith, Sarah Lavelle, Fiona MacIntyre, and all. At Atria, I thank Greer Hendricks, Sybil Pincus, Annette Corkey, Suzanne Fass, and Caroline Stearns.

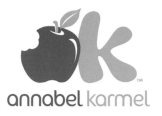

annabel karmel

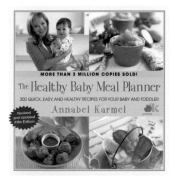

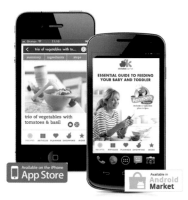

As your child grows. . .

Let Annabel guide you through the next stage with The Healthy Baby Meal Planner. Packed full of useful advice and recipes, you will find that this bestselling, classic cookbook is the perfect guide to preparing healthy, tasty meals for your child.

You can also download Annabel's recently updated App, Annabel's Essential Guide To Feeding Your Baby & Toddler, for lots of new, nutritious, and easy recipes plus exclusive video content showing you everything from food preparation to step-by-step guides. You will also find two episodes of Annabel's Kitchen, perfect for keeping little ones entertained!